How To Fight Cancer And Win

How To Fight Cancer And Win

*Scientific Guidelines and documented
facts for the successful treatment
and prevention of cancer and other
related health problems.*

William L. Fischer

Fischer Publishing Corporation
Canfield, Ohio 44406

Dedication

I believe the preventive approach to the killing diseases is the one best hope for the future health of people every- where. You won't find a 'miracle pill' anywhere that can magically conquer cancer overnight - not now, and probably not ever. But many important and scientifically documented strides have been taken recently in the fast-growing field of Preventive Medicine. All the preventives that have been proven in research to have sound merit are presented for your thoughtful consideration within the pages of this book. I also point an accusing finger at some of the commercial interests who are feeding the public known carcinogens by the means of some misleading advertising. What you don't know *can* hurt you.

I dedicate this book to the prevention and eradication of cancer and the other killing degenerative diseases that pervade our nation and the westernized societies of the world today.

Disclaimer

This book is informational only and should not be considered as a substitute for consultation with a duly-licensed medical doctor. Any attempt to diagnose and treat an illness should come under the direction of a physician. The author is not himself a medical doctor and does not purport to offer medical advice, make diagnoses, prescribe remedies for specific medical conditions or substitute for medical consultation.

While all case histories in this book are true, names have been changed or shortened to protect the identities of the persons described.

TABLE OF CONTENTS

Chapter 4
DIET AS A WEAPON

Chapter 5
THE IMPORTANCE OF DIETARY FATS

Chapter 6
THE MIRACLE OF LINSEED OIL

Chapter 11
LITTLE-KNOWN CANCER PREVENTIVES & SOME AVOIDABLE CARCINOGENS

Chapter 12
HEALTHY LIVING

Chapter 13
GETTING BACK TO BASIC NUTRITION

Chapter 14
EMINENT DOCTORS & ALTERNATIVE CANCER
TREATMENTS TODAY

Chapter 15
FOREWARNED IS FOREARMED

About The Author

William L. Fischer has been involved in medicine, health care and natural healing for over thirty years. After working with several of the largest pharmaceutical manufacturers in his native Germany, he founded his own health company in Heidelberg. Later, he moved to the United States and began publishing books on natural healing. To obtain the most comprehensive information available, his research has taken him around the world to such diverse places such as Iran, The Far East, Europe and Egypt to study natural healing techniques and practices of other cultures. He is the author of over a dozen books including:

• Chelation Therapy • Throw Away Your Eyeglasses and Contact Lenses • The Miracle Healing Power Through Nature's Pharmacy • How To Survive In the Hospital • Hidden Secrets of Super Perfect Health at Any Age, Books I and II • The Romace of Creative Healthy Cookery • The Youth Renewal Revolution • Secrets To Healthy Eyes • Breakthroughs In Arthritis • Secrets To A Healthy Heart and Low Cholesterol • Miraculous Breakthroughs for Prostate and Impotency Problems • Eye Secrets To Better Sight • How To Fight Cancer and Win.

Foreword

In modern alternative medicine we have found it is absolutely necessary to treat the entire person - his emotions, attitudes, nutrition, immune system, inner spirituality and relationships - in order to bring about inner peace, stress relief and healing. This is how a patient reaches a new balance of health, and symptoms and discomfort simply disappear. He will be cured of the serious health problem or problems that exist when the patient is first seen.

As a Medical Doctor and Internationally-known opthalmologist whose studies in eye problems have been conducted at clinics and universities through Europe and the U.S., allow me to quickly outline how this natural, alternative approach came to us. Hippocrates, "the Father of Medicine," introduced holistic concepts - treating not only symptoms and specific body parts, but the entire body. His theory was expanded upon by the great Roman physician Galen. Several hundred years later, a royal doctor named Paracelsus introduced the concept of a human immune system and natural antibiotics.

Paracelsus served several royal families in Austria and Hungary. His theory was vividly portrayed in a folk tale handed down to us through several generations. Once, while Paracelsus was riding in his carriage through the countryside, an excited peasant man flagged down the coachman and asked to speak to the famous doctor.

A fellow in a nearby village had just been run down by a heavy cart. Paracelsus agreed to examine the injured man where he lay in the street. He found no broken bones, but a deep cut in the man's thigh was bleeding profusely.

Then, much to the onlookers' dismay, the regally robed physician pointed to a nearby pile of steaming-fresh horse droppings. "Pick it up, and spread it on the wound," he told a bystander. The man obeyed, but the people mumbled among themselves. They didn't understand the technique, but Paracelsus did - the dung contained immune and antibiotic qualities taken from the insides of the horse who left it behind. Its presence would help heal the wound itself, while triggering the man's own immunities to fight infection.

The doctor left some instructions on binding the wound, and went on his way. The villagers continued to stand and watch, expecting to hear the injured man utter his last words. After about 20 minutes the dung was removed and the wound bandaged. But not before the villagers saw the results: a cut that had already stopped bleeding, lost its swelling and begun to knit together.

Although I won't advocate piling manure on your cuts and bruises, I feel this illustrates my point: alternative medical methods that operate outside accepted orthodox treatments really can work. They are now becoming recognized and accepted by the general public. Even the most fearful diseases, like cancer, tumors and glaucoma, are being successfully treated using these "unorthodox" methods.

Paracelsus has many modern successors whose methods take a "whole body" approach. They include Dr. Edward Bach, Herbert Shelton, and Paavo Airola; and more recently Gerald Jampolsky, Leo Buscaglia and Eric Siegal. These doctors and teachers are conscious of the great influence of natural foods, quality relationships and personal spirituality can have on bodily health.

Their findings are popping up even in high-tech teaching hospitals, where young doctors are taught the basics of natural organic nutrition, visualization and bio-feedback therapies and the importance of mental attitudes in healing the entire body. Several of these methods, therapies and techniques are described in this book. As odd as some may appear, they are usually based in nature, and use your body's own healing mechanisms to attack the diseases that might otherwise overcome you.

Alternative methods outside of orthodox medical approaches are being more and more recognized and accepted by the general public. These methods, especially in serious conditions such as tumors, cancers, etc., are getting good results and cures.

The author of this book isn't a doctor, but he is a recognized author and authority on natural nutrition and health. Many of the treatments outlined here work very well also in conjunction with orthodox cancer treatments like radiation, chemotherapy or surgery.

And remember, too, that your health is your own, to ignore or care for throughout a lifetime. Not even a doctor can undo the damage that years of neglect or abuse can cost your body. I hope you read this in good health; if not, I hope its sound advice can help you regain what was lost.

Leslie H. Salov, M.D., O.D., Ph. D.

Preface

Cancer is the second leading cause of death in the United States. In 1985 alone, cancer claimed the lives of 462,000 Americans. Of this number, 161,700 cancer deaths (35 percent) are believed to be attributable to dietary factors. Every bite of food that enters the body plays a key role in determining the degree of health we enjoy.

Dietary studies around the world have shown that excessive intake of the wrong kind of fats, particularly when coupled with an inadequate consumption of fiber, results in a higher incidence of certain cancers. Research shows that a deficiency of certain important vitamins and minerals in the diet fosters the development of cancerous tumors. It is entirely possible that simply making some sweeping changes in the national diet could dramatically reduce the number of lives lost to cancer every year.

The National Cancer Institute now recognizes the important part that the correct diet can play in an effective cancer preventive program. In their report entitled, "Diet, Nutrition, and Cancer," the NCI names healthy foods and zeros in on suspect foods. *In How to Fight Cancer And Win,* William L. Fischer details the recommendations encompassed by the NCI report with an explanation of how these foods work physiologically. He also deals with the best diet recommendations coming out of important world-wide research. This information is a real eye-opener and you'll learn some astounding facts.

William Fischer has also presented the case for bee pollen, a powerful cancer preventive, as succinctly as possible. Considering the mountain of scientific documentation that exists on the medicinal benefits of what many call "nature's perfect food," this material alone is the result of many long hours of concentrated research.

The author's main purpose in writing this book is to alert the general public to important advances in preventive medicine. A series of measures based on present medical knowledge in the fields of nutrition, oncogenes, viruses, immunology, detection, diagnosis, treatment, rehabilitation and prevention have been targeted by health authorities with the avowed aim of reducing the number of new cancer cases by

50 percent by the year 2000. In order to achieve this goal, dietary treatments should be implemented in conjunction with, when necessary, other cancer therapeutic modalities, including surgery, radiation, chemotherapy, and biological response modifier programs, all described in this book.

Although the main purpose of this book is to encourage a preventive approach to all health disorders, including cancer, you'll find a detailed review of what's going on in current research, plus both the old and new treatments favored by orthodox medicine. I personally favor preventive medicine as being the only viable approach to conquering the killer diseases forever. Once you have read through this material and understand the importance of making the necessary changes in your lifestyle, I believe you will agree.

Suffice it to say that, within these pages you will find the first comprehensive, consolidated, and concise material covering the entire scope of the cancer problem ever written especially for the layperson. It is presented in an easy-to-read and easy-to-understand manner. You won't need a dictionary at your elbow to decipher this book. All in all, this book should serve its intended audience admirably. I urge you to take this information under close consideration. It is entirely possible that your future health and happiness are at stake.

Amar Makheja, Ph.D.
Doctor of Biochemistry
The George Washington University School of Medicine
Washington, D.C.

A Letter From The Author

Dear Friends,

While I was abroad doing some of the research for this book, I had the good fortune to secure some important material written by the great international oncologist, Dr. Hans Nieper. His work is well known and highly respected all over the world. In fact, I have it on good authority that Dr. Nieper's writings on cancer treatment and prevention were consulted when our own U.S. President Ronald Reagan underwent successful treatment last year for cancerous polyps discovered in his colon. Many of Dr. Nieper's revolutionary findings are reviewed in this book.

In another highlight of my month-long trip, I was favored with a great courtesy by Dr. Johanna Budwig. Dr. Budwig was kind enough to spare some of her valuable time to meet with me personally. This amazing 79 year old woman has the verve, vitality, and energy of a lady in her 50s. Although I had read much of her incredible work, I was impressed all over again by both the woman herself and the documented cures of cancer and other debilitating and killing diseases she has accomplished with a program of simple nutrition. I personally talked with some of the people she has helped when orthodox medicine could offer no successful treatment.

Dr. Budwig shared her research on linseed oil with me and I brought back the chemical and biological documentation on just how this medicinal fat works miracles within the human body, presented for your consideration in Chapter VII. Dr. Budwig is a true humanitarian in the largest sense of the word.

All in all, this was a highly successful research mission. I was very gratified at the reception I received at the hands of the many, many scientists and specialists in the various areas of expertise we examined for presentation in this book. I think we have managed to cull the best from the best minds around the world working on the cancer problem.

I was particularly struck by the informed health-consciousness of the ordinary citizen abroad. Although many times I was invited to break bread with friends, both old and new, I often took a solitary meal in the local restaurant where I was stopping in Europe. A great many of these establishments routinely place small dishes of what I first took to be the usual condiments on the table in front of the patron. I was both astounded and very pleased to find that these dishes contained raw seeds of every description! The diner could choose from among linseeds (flaxseed), poppy seeds, pumpkin seeds, chia seeds, raw almonds, and on and on. It was delightful to be able to sprinkle a selection of seeds on a salad, use some to dress a vegetable, or simply crunch and munch a handful of health while waiting to be served.

When I first ran across this little 'seed buffet' on my table, I thought it was an isolated instance and that the restaurant owner was a health buff. But, as time went on, I found that this healthful nicety was really quite commonplace. I finally struck up a conversation with the proprietor of one of the restaurants serving seeds and questioned him. He told me that it was the result of popular demand and had been established a few years back. His regular customers expected to be served a selection of seeds. He went on to say that he had tried to discontinue the practice two years ago and found that his customers complained or went elsewhere to eat.

Some informed and knowledgeable U.S. restauranteurs have adopted this idea and serve raw seeds along with the greens and vegetables in prominent display on their salad bars. As more and more Americans make known their desire to 'eat right,' this healthy practice could sweep the country!

To your very good health,
William L. Fischer

Chapter I

Cancer Explained

What It Is & What It Does

WHAT IT IS — Cancer in man is a group of related diseases (over 100) which may develop in any part of the body. Cancer can strike anyone of any age, but comes more frequently as we get older. One death in every five in the U.S. comes from cancer. Statistics show that over 66 million Americans now living will eventually develop cancer. Cancer occurs in just about three out of every four families in the United States and it kills more children between the ages of 3 and 14 than any other disease.

But a diagnosis of cancer is not necessarily a death sentence. Dr. Vincent T. DeVita, Jr., Director of the National Cancer Institute, says, "The American people are unduly pessimistic about what happens to them when they have cancer. Truly, half the cancers in this country are curable." Statistics from the N.C.I. show steady progress against this most-feared of all diseases. In the 1930s, less than 20 percent of cancer victims survived for five years. By the 1940s, the five-year rate of survival had grown to 25 percent. Today, over 50 percent of diagnosed cancer patients survive to reach the magic number of five years. Children have fared even better. At least 60 percent are expected to be among those surviving for five years.

WHAT IT DOES — How does this killer operate? In brief, *cancer is the uncontrolled and disorderly multiplication of abnormal cells which form* a malignant *tumor* (neoplasm) that

1

is usually identified medically as a *carcinoma* or *sarcoma,* depending on what part of the body is involved. The main difference between *benign* and *malignant* tumors is that benign tumors are usually enclosed within a capsule composed of a membrane of connective tissue. Benign tumors don't spread and degenerative cell changes are much less frequent than in malignant tumors.

But a cancerous cell operates outside natural law. Cancer destroys life by invading an essential organ where it grows out of control. When it expands to the point where the organ can no longer carry on its essential function, death inevitably follows. Dr. Lance Liotta, Chief of the NCI's Laboratory of Pathology, explains, "Cancer invasion and metastasis (spreading) is the main cause of treatment failure. That is really what kills the patient in most cases."

The human body is a gigantic collection of cells. Cells and the products of cells make up all the tissues and organs of the body. All bodily functions are carried on by cells. Cells of one tissue differ from those of other tissues, depending on what function they perform. The chromosomes contained in the nucleus of each cell carry the programming that determines how the cell will function in the body.

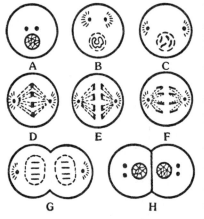

Normal Cell Division

Four phases of mitotic division in a cell having four chromosomes. A, B, C, Changes in the centrosome and nucleus during prophase. D, Metaphase. E, F, Anaphase. G, H, Telophase.

New cells develop only from preexisting cells and come into being by a process called *mitosis,* or cell division. During mitosis, the cell's chromosomes divide and move to opposite sides of the original cell. Upon completion of the last of the four phases of mitosis, each of the two new daughter cells is an exact duplicate of the original cell, complete with a full set of programmed chromosomes that tell it what to do and how to function.

ONCOGENES — This term comes from the Greek word 'onkos,' or tumor, and signifies a gene with the potential to cause a cancerous tumor. Packed into each and every cell in our body are upwards of 50,000 bits of information called genes. Genes comprise the genetic code for all parts of our bodies. Among the 50,000 genes present in each cell, science has identified about 20 different proto-oncogenes in perfectly normal genetic material. This means that every single one of us carries proto-oncogenes capable of developing into cancer.

Since proto-oncogenes are present in all normal cells, the question is *what turns them on?* Why do some unfortunate individuals develop cancer while others, even those in the same household, do not? Researchers are working overtime to target the triggers. Certain external factors (including chemicals, viruses, exposure to radiation) are being investigated because of their ability to cause gene-mutations. In connection with a Milan, Italy cancer research institute, the NCI (National Cancer Institute, Bethesda, Maryland) has conducted studies which indicate that a mutagenic agent can cause a normal cell to turn cancerous.

Since the exciting news that oncogenes have been identified, scientists all over the world are now investigating two different theories: (1) Can just one activated oncogene produce cancer?, or (2) Must multiple oncogenes be activated to produce cancer?

A cautious dissenting voice protesting the enthusiasm expressed by many scientists comes from Professor Peter H. Duesberg, Department of Molecular Biology, University of California, Berkeley. Publishing in the May 10th, 1985 issue of *Science,* Professor Duesberg says, "Despite the popularity of these hypotheses, it is pointed out here that there is as yet no convincing evidence that activated proto-oncogenes are necessary, much less sufficient, for carcinogenesis."

However, independent but related laboratory experiments undertaken by three different groups appear to confirm the theory that mutated genes do develop into cancer. Studies conducted by Robert A. Weinberg, Massachusetts Institute of Technology, and R.F. Newbold and R.W. Overell of the Institute of Cancer Research, Buckinghamshire, England, and H. Earl

3

Ruley, of the Cold Spring Harbor Laboratory in New York, support the hypothesis that at least two agents are required for a malignancy to develop. These scientists all produced cancer in their respective laboratories by treating normal genes with two carcinogenic agents.

Weinberg reported that a single cancer gene does not turn normal rat embryo cells cancerous, but that pairs of cancer genes do. Ruley's research confirmed that pairs of cancerous genes produce a malignancy, but a lone cancer gene does not. The British researchers found that newborn hamster skin cells became cancerous when treated with a carcinogenic chemical and one cancer gene, but not when treated singly with one or the other.

All in all, now that science has identified proto-oncogenes in the genetic material stored in our cells and is hot on the trail of the triggers that turn them on, certainly some optimism is justified. Once we know what turns them on, science has a good chance of developing a method of turning them off. In the meantime, avoiding known mutagenic agents just makes good sense. (See Chapter 4.)

When examined under a microscope, early cancer cells look very much like the original healthy cells from which they originated. Indeed, they may function *almost* normally for a while, with little or no symptoms to give you a clue they are planning to wreak havoc within your body. This is one reason why early detection is difficult. The body automatically repairs cellular damage in an ongoing process, but when enough harm is caused to the cell's DNA (deoxyribonucleic acid) programming, it is turned into an active oncogene and cell division goes out of control. The DNA fights damage coming from many sources, including carcinogenic (cancer-causing) chemicals in water, food, and the polluted environment, plus unavoidable cosmic radiation, ultraviolet light from the sun, radiation from diagnostic x-rays, viral infections, and random genetic alterations. On top of all that, smokers pollute both themselves and the air we all breathe with the documented carcinogens in tobacco smoke.

As the DNA begins to lose the battle and the disease progresses, the cancer cells become increasingly abnormal in appearance, structure, and function. Chromosomes in malignant cells undergoing division become oversized and many exhibit additional abnormalities showing up in a large number of different sizes and shapes. A single cell with active oncogenes divides into two abnormal cells, then four, then eight, and so on. Each cell

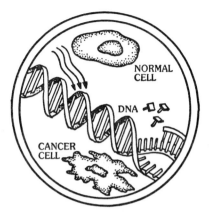

**The Development of
A Cancerous Cell**

divides until a malignant lump (tumor) begins to form. After a period of time, which varies considerably depending on the type of cancer, the malignant cells can no longer be recognized as daughters of the original healthy cell tissue.

A comforting thought comes from Dr. Curtis Harris, Chief of the National Cancer Institute's Laboratory of Human Carcinogenesis. Dr. Harris points out that a normal cell must go through at least four distinct steps to become cancerous. As you read through these steps, outlined below, please be very much aware that we can exert considerable control over Step One.

Step One   A carcinogen (dietary factors, chemical pollutants, tobacco smoke) turns on an oncogene, the first step in preparing to make the cell cancerous.

Step Two   The cell is now medically termed *precancerous* and begins to grow more actively than a normal cell, but it is not yet a true cancer cell. (If precancerous cells are promptly identified in nonessential tissue, a physician may opt for early removal of the involved cells to prevent steps three and four from occurring.)

Step Three   If identification is not made and no intervening measures are instituted, another muta-
tion may occur. When this happens, the
precancerous cell evolves into true cancer.

Step Four   At this point, the cell's DNA programming
has become genetically unstable and muta-
tion progresses rapidly, resulting in the
development of a malignant tumor.

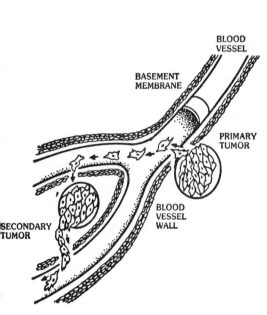

Metastasis

If their wild multiplication is not
checked, the cancer cells will
freely invade and destroy
neighboring tissue. A particular
danger is that the malignant
cells can hitch a ride and travel
through the bloodstream or
lymphatic system to establish a
cancer colony in another part
of the body. The medical term
for the ability of a malignancy
to spring up in another part of
the body is called *metastasis*.
In order to spread, cancer cells
must break through the thin
layer of membrane (basement
lamina) which protects all
tissue from invasion. Once
cancer cells have broken into
the bloodsteam (or have
invaded a lymph node), they
are carried along by the blood
(or lymphatic fluid) until they
become lodged in a new area.
There they again tunnel
through the protective membrane where they divide and
multiply until a new cancer is
formed.

6

How Cancer Spreads Through The Body

Although most cancer cells die en route to other parts of the body, enough survive the turbulence of the bloodstream and the body's immunological defenses to reach the lungs, brain, liver and kidneys. Those organs filter blood through tiny capillaries, which trap the cancer cells. They then grow into secondary tumors, which crowd out functioning organs.

BRAIN METASTASIS
SPREADS THROUGH ARTERY
SPREADS THROUGH VEIN
LYMPH NODE
LUNG METASTASIS
LIVER METASTASIS
PRIMARY TUMOR
STOMACH CANCER
OVARY METASTASIS

Routes of spread of cancer of the prostate to adjacent tissues: 1. bladder; 2. abdominal cavity; 3. rectum; 4. anal sphincters; 5. urethra. Early cancer of the prostate does not usually cause symptoms of bladder obstruction and the best hope of early discovery is rectal examination at intervals advised by a physician.

PROSTATE

The deep lymphatic vessels and glands of the abdomen and pelvis.

Kidney
Lumbar glands
Sacral glands
Internal iliac glands
Rectum
Bladder
Deep lymphatics of penis
Testicle

In some cases of malignant disease, these glands become enormously enlarged.

(Sacral glands) These and the internal iliac glands are affected in malignant disease of the *bladder*, *rectum* or *uterus*.

Cancer spreads throughout the body by piercing the protective membrances enclosing all tissue. It then enters the bloodstream or lymphatic system. As primary cancer cells become lodged in the tiny capillaries feeding vital organs or in the lymph passageways, they form secondary tumors. As these secondary tumors multiply and divide, they begin to encroach on the host organ. Eventually, if allowed to proliferate, the organ is so infiltrated by the tumor that it can no longer perform its essential function.

7

WHAT ARE MY CHANCES?

The table below, from NCI statistics, shows a wide variance in the five-year survival and mortality rates for the major types of cancer. There's even a variance in your chances depending on whether you're male or female, black or white. These figures are based on the number of cancer cases per 100,000 persons. Look them over carefully. Then pay close attention to the documented preventive measures you'll find in the pages of this book

NCI SUMMARY OF INCIDENCE, MORTALITY, & 5-YEAR SURVIVAL RATES

Site/Type	Incidence		Mortality		% Surviving 5-Yrs	
	White	Black	White	Black	White	Black
Breast	85.6	71.9	26.6	26.3	75	63
Bladder	15.4	8.6	3.9	3.8	74	50
Cervix	8.8	20.2	3.2	8.8	68	63
Esophagus	2.9	11.5	2.6	9.2	5	3
Larynx	4.6	6.6	1.3	2.5	67	59
Lung	81.0	119.0	70.7	91.4	13	10
Multiple myeloma	3.4	7.9	2.4	5.0	24	27
Pancreas	8.9	13.6	8.6	11.0	3	3
Prostate	75.1	120.3	21.0	43.9	69	59
Rectum	15.0	11.7	3.5	3.5	49	37
Stomach	2.9	11.5	2.6	9.2	5	5
Uterus	25.1	13.4	2.0	2.9	88	57

WHAT CAUSES CANCER?

In the past ten years alone, science has come a long way in understanding the way cancer develops and what triggers the mutations that cause a normal cell to turn cancerous. The

8

National Cancer Institute says emphatically that many cancers can be prevented by making appropriate changes in our lifestyle. There are a number of areas where we have full control. By making the right choices, we can exercise a preventive effect against cancer.

ENVIRONMENT — The man-made chemical carcinogens which pollute the food chain and are present in our drinking water and air are largely unavoidable. Even the NCI notes that cleaning up the environment will require broad social actions or system changes to achieve effective controls. But you can ask your doctor if that x-ray is really necessary, and you can work with your employer to reduce your exposure to carcinogens which may be a part of your occupational hazard.

In fact, the NCI has exposure to occupational carcinogens as a preventable health hazard. Plans on the drawing board include educating both employers and employees in certain industries (asbestos, benzene, anilene dye) to the dangers and working with these companies to develop stringent safety standards. Incidentally, you should know that smokers who work in these industries are increasing their risk of developing cancer 50 times over.

GENETIC FACTORS — You have no control over the genes you were born with, but people born into a 'cancer-prone' family can still adopt healthy habits and have a good chance of escaping the disease.

LIFESTYLE CHOICES

The NCI points out that we have control over many factors which comprise a large part of our lifestyles. These factors include eliminating the use of tobacco, selecting preventive foods, eliminating suspect foods, reducing our exposure to sunlight, adopting healthy sex habits (and choosing a healthy partner), and practicing good personal hygiene.

SMOKING — Over 130,000 people die needlessly of cancer every year simply because they refuse to give up smoking tobacco. NCI statistics reveal that about 30 percent of all cancer deaths are directly attributable to smoking. It is a fact that those who smoke two or more packs of the 'cancer sticks' daily have a lung cancer death rate twenty-five times higher than non-smokers. In 1986, data shows that lung cancer may exceed breast cancer as the leading cause of cancer death among U.S. women for the first time. Since the early 1950s, lung cancer rates have increased 256 percent among women and 172 percent among men. In spite of the scientific evidence targeting the carcinogens in tobacco smoke as a cause of cancer, known and publicized for over twenty years, there are still close to half a million Americans (approximately one out of every three adults) who still puff away their lives — one breath at a time.

Smoking tobacco is the prime cause of both lung and laryngeal cancers, a major cause of oral and esophageal cancers, and contributes heavily to the development of bladder, kidney, and pancreatic cancers. In addition, some research indicates that a relationship between smoking and stomach, cervical, and liver cancers exists. The risk of developing cancer rises with the amount of tobacco smoked, the amount of tar exposure, and the number of years smoking has continued. Here are the frightening statistics:

Lung Cancer: In 1981 (the last year for which figures are available), 106,389 people died in the U.S. from lung cancer. Over 90 percent of lung cancer in men and 77 percent in women can be traced to cigarette smoking. When you tally up these percentages, you find that over 90,000 men and women died as a result of smoking. If you use tobacco, the odds are over-whelmingly against you.

Laryngeal Cancer: The risk of developing cancer of the larynx is 20 to 30 times higher for smokers than for nonsmokers. The major cause of laryngeal cancer is smoking. About 75 percent of the laryngeal cancer in men is attributable to tobacco smoking, compared to approximately 43 percent in women.

Oral Cancer: Projections of the mortality rate of oral cancer in tobacco users range up to thirteen times greater for smokers than for nonsmokers. This also applies to users of 'smokeless tobacco,' i.e. chewing tobacco and snuff.

Esophageal Cancer: The risk of death from esophageal cancer has been shown to be up to twelve times higher for smokers than for nonsmokers.

Other Cancers: Approximately 40 percent of the cases of *pancreatic cancer* are attributable to smoking. The risk factor for pancreatic cancer for smokers is twice that for nonsmokers. About 56 percent of the incidence of *bladder cancer* can be traced to smoking. The risk of a smoker developing *bladder cancer* is up to seven times higher than the nonsmoker. And smokers carry five times the risk of dying from *kidney cancer* as nonsmokers.

You Can't Beat the Odds: If you took your life savings to Las Vegas and played the tables against odds like these, you'd end up bankrupt. These are heavy odds to have working against you. The Surgeon General of the United States says, *"Cigarette smoking is the chief, single, avoidable cause of death in our society and the most important public health issue of our time."*

THE DIETARY FACTORS — Figures from the National Cancer Institute show that approximately 35 percent of all cancers can be attributed to dietary imbalances. Since the early 1900s, we have steadily *increased* our consumption of meat, poultry, fish, dairy products, refined sugars and sweeteners, fats and oils, and processed fruits and vegetables. We have steadily *reduced* our consumption of whole grain products, potatoes, fresh fruits and vegetables, and eggs. Let's face it. We've gotten lazy. We *like* our overprocessed chemical-saturated convenience foods.

But a vast number of studies show that excessive fat intake, inadequate dietary fiber, and a deficiency of important micronutrients (vitamins and minerals) are related to higher rates of certain cancers. (In Chapter 4, you will find an extensive review of what foods should be on the menu and what you'd be better off eliminating.) Dietary insufficiencies and excesses are associated with cancers of the gastrointestinal tract (including the esophagus, stomach, colon, rectum, pancreas, and liver), plus sex and hormone-specific sites (such as the breast, prostate, ovaries, and endometrium). Dietary factors also play a part in the development of cancers of the respiratory system and the urinary tract.

Figures Don't Lie: What we want to bring home to you here is that it's up to you to incorporate the appropriate preventive measures into your lifestyle. You don't have to smoke. And you control what you serve for dinner. The table below, prepared with hard data from the National Cancer Institute, shows very graphically that simply by eliminating tobacco and eating correctly we can reduce cancer mortality by 65 percent. And those are *good* odds to have working in your favor.

CAUSES OF CANCER DEATH

Factors Identified	Percent of Cancer Deaths
Dietary Factors	35%
Tobacco Use	30%
Sexual Behavior/Reproductive Systems	7%
Occupational Hazards	4%
Alcohol	3%
Geophysical Factors	3%
Pollution (water/food/environment)	2%
Industrial Products	1%
Medicines & Medical Procedures	1%

EARLY IDENTIFICATION VITAL

ELIMINATING THE HANDICAP — Early identification is the single greatest problem in the medical treatment of a malignancy. If cancers stayed where they began and didn't grow and spread, most malignant tumors could be successfully treated. For instance, in the case of a localized cancer, the five-year survival rate is well over 80 percent. However, if the exact same type of tumor invades the lymph nodes, which have pathways all over the body, the five-year survival rate drops to around 32 percent. Only 1.2 percent of persons with metastasized (spreading) cancers survive for five years.

Quite obviously, the medical treatment of an early *prime* (original) cancer is many times more successful, and less drastic, than the treatment required for cancer which has

12

spread (metastasized) from its original site to other parts of the body. Many scientists believe more than half of all cancers can be completely cured if identified in their early stages. Early detection and prompt effective treatment is essential.

DIAGNOSTIC TECHNIQUES

EARLY DETECTION — There are a number of common medical techniques which allow doctors to detect and diagnose an early malignancy. Even more non-invasive diagnostic aids are being developed by scientists around the world. Very soon, a biopsy, in which the surgeon takes a cutting of suspect tissue for microscopic examination, may be a thing of the past. Here's a quick review of the most common methods of detection.

Cervical Cancer: One of the easiest and most effective techniques for detecting cervical cancer in women is the Pap test. By examining the cells naturally sloughed off by the uterus, the physician can identify a potentially dangerous precancerous condition, or an existing malignancy, and initiate prompt treatment. Data shows that death from cervical cancer is on the decline, but is still far from a rare occurrence, especially among black women.

Bladder Cancer: Cells that are shed by the bladder into the urine may indicate the presence of early bladder cancer. Certain groups at high risk of developing bladder cancer, such as workers in the aniline-dye industry, are routinely screened by this method.

Breast Cancer: Mammography, a special x-ray technique, can detect breast cancers as tiny as two-tenths (0.2) of an inch, much too small to be felt. Another new procedure, *thermography,* records the heat patterns of the breast and allows the physician to note the pattern characteristic of early cancer. It is important to note here that statistics show that regular breast examinations, including screening with mammography, have led to a reduction in deaths due to breast cancer, not only over the short term, but in the long run as well. A survey conducted by the NCI revealed that only one out of every five women surveyed reported ever having had a mammogram.

13

The NCI is out to change these statistics. The experts say that annual screening would result in a 30 percent reduction in breast cancer mortality.

One final note: After all the controversy over the relationship of oral contraceptives to breast cancer, data coming from an extensive Swedish study and Norwegian study (as published in the prestigious British publication, *Lancet,* September 1986) appears to be conclusive. We quote from pertinent passages: "We found no statistically significant association between the use of oral contraceptives for 7 completed years or less with premenopausal breast cancer. However, our data for the long-term use of oral contraceptives beyond 7 years and particularly for 12 years or more are suggestive of an association with an increased risk of premenopausal breast cancer. The duration of oral contraceptive use before the first full-term pregnancy and the total duration of use correlated strongly in our series." In other words, young women who use oral contraceptives before their first-term pregnancy are just as much at risk of developing breast cancer as are women who take the pill for 12 years or more. If you refuse to give up this popular form of birth control (and many of you will prefer to take your chances), it is doubly important that you regularly monitor your breasts for lumps and have regular screenings by your physician.

Colorectal Cancer: Unfortunately, the early detection of colorectal cancer by means of a proctoscopic examination has not been popular among the general public and few physicians employ this means of examination on a routine basis. If you value your life and health, you might want to consider having an annual proctoscopic exam after the age of forty.

Sam Shapiro, B.S., past director of the Health Services Research & Development Center (Baltimore, Maryland) and Professor Emeritus, School of Public Health, Johns Hopkins University (Baltimore, Maryland) points out that "There is a strong conviction in many circles that a public education program, accompanied by elevated professional attention, is needed to increase knowledge about risk factors and receptivity to messages about diet, improve responsiveness to symptoms, and increase the frequency of proctoscopy performance as part of general physical examinations starting for those in the middle years of life."

Lung Cancer: A technique similar to the Pap test can be used to verify a suspected lung cancer long before it is large enough to appear on an x-ray. A microscopic examination of cells taken from the surface of the oral cavity can assist in identifying early mouth and throat cancer.

Oral Cancer: You might not even be aware that your dentist looks for the tell-tale early warning signs of oral cancer while he's poking around your mouth with his instruments. Oral cancer cases are on the increase. In 1985, close to 30,000 new cases were discovered in the U.S., more than double the cases reported in 1970. Science says that tobacco (especially cigarettes and chewing tobacco), alcohol, syphilis, and bad oral hygiene are the major contributing factors. In addition, new studies indicate that the herpes simplex virus and a chronic iron deficiency increase oral cancer risk.

Your dentist is an able diagnostician of oral cancer. But the problem is that we don't always see our dentist often enough. The elderly, at high risk of developing oral cancer, go to their medical doctor six times more often than they go to the dentist. Statistics show that half of those age 65 or older have not seen a dentist in five or more years. For those age 65 or older who wear dentures, more than seventy percent have not seen a dentist in five years or more.

In every 100,000 persons, 7.5 will die from oral cancer. Probably because more men than women chew tobacco and drink, the breakdown is 5.6 men in every 100,000, compared to 1.9 women. Three-quarters of these deaths are in persons 55 years of age and older. The five-year survival rate is low (30-35%), possibly because half of the oral cancers have metastasized before being discovered.

Drs. G.T. Chiodo, T. Eigner, and D.I. Rosenstein, publishing in *Postgraduate Medicine* (August 1986) believe that once primary care physicians routinely screen for oral cancer, survival rates will improve. They say, "Prognosis improves vastly when the lesion is detected and treated early. One study has demonstrated a 64 percent five-year survival rate for patients with oral cancer that was diagnosed before regional lymph node involvement versus a 15 percent five-year survival rate for patients whose lesions were diagnosed after metastasis. By including an oral cancer examination in routine physical examination of patients, the physician and public health nurse can increase the likelihood of early detection of oral cancer." In the meantime, the bottom line is that you should see your dentist twice a year, and not just to have your teeth cleaned either.

LOOKING AHEAD

The National Cancer Institute has developed a comprehensive program aimed at substantially reducing the number of cancer cases in the nation by the year 2000. A detailed plan entitled *Cancer Control — Objectives for the Nation — 1985 to 2000* has already been implemented. The following table summarizes these objectives and what the NCI is doing about them. The following statement comes from this landmark NCI report: *"On the basis of current knowledge alone, the NCI estimates that, at a minimum, 30,000 lives could be saved in the year 2000 if Americans would modify their dietary habits."* The key to the success (or failure) of this grand goal is you and me and every citizen of the U.S. We have the knowledge to make it work. All we have to do is follow the plan and incorporate these recommendations in our lives.

MEDICAL PROCEDURES

TYPE OF CANCER DETERMINES TREATMENT — The successful medical treatment of cancer requires the complete removal or destruction of all malignant tissue. The first line of defense is surgery. For surgery to provide a cure for cancer, the operation must be performed before the malignancy has spread into organs and tissues that sustain life.

The choice of medical treatment against cancer is governed by the type, location, and size of the tumor at the time of diagnosis. Surgery, radiation, chemotherapy, drug and hormone treatments, laser and heat therapies, interferon, anti-

THE NCI CANCER CONTROL OBJECTIVES

Action	Target	Rationale	Year 2000 Objectives	Estimated Death Reduction
Prevention	Smoking	The relationship between smoking and cancer has been scientifically established.	Reduce percentage of adults who smoke from 34% (in 1983) to 15% or less. Reduce percentage of youths who smoke by age 20 from 36% (in 1983) to 15% or less.	8 to 15%
	Diet	Research shows that high-fat low-fiber consumption may increase risk for various cancers. Studies have persuaded the NCI to recommend an increase in fiber. New research is underway to verify the relationships and test the impact on cancer incidence.	Reduce average consumption of fat from 38% to 30% or less of total calories. Increase average consumption of fiber from 8-12 grams to 20-30 grams daily.	8%
Screening	Breast	The effectiveness of breast screening in reducing mortality has been scientifically established.	Increase percentage of women aged 50-70 who have an annual breast exam coupled with mammography from 45% to 80% for physical exam and 15% for mammography.	3%
	Cervix	The effectiveness of cervical screening in reducing mortality has been scientifically established.	Increase percentage of women who have a Pap smear every 3 years from 79% (ages 20-39) to 90% and from 57% (ages 40-70) to 80%.	3%
Treatment	Put research results into practice.	NCI review of certain trials and data shows that (for certain cancer sites) mortality is greater than experienced in clinical trials.	Increase adoption of state-of-the-art treatment.	10 to 14%
Treatment		With accelerated gains in state-of-the-art treatment.		26%
Total Range of Mortality (Death-Rate) Reduction by Year 2000				**25 to 50%**

bodies, and the special knowledge of oncogenes, are some of the cancer-fighting methods available to the treating physician.

Often the busy physician is unable to take the time needed to really sit down with a patient and explain what the projected therapy is designed to do and what to expect. But a thorough understanding of the procedure goes a long way toward reassuring the patient and helps make the treatment a thousand times more bearable.

In this book, under the heading of *Scientific Discoveries,* we examine the various medical treatments currently in use against cancer, or just over the horizon. In non-technical language, we explain exactly how the newest methods work, how well they work (or don't work), and how they affect the body. We report on the latest developments in cancer research and let you in on the progress the scientists are making.

In the segment entitled *Nutritional & Holistic Treatments,* you are introduced to certain common nutrients that many authorities believe can strengthen the body against cancer. We examine the macrobiotic diet and explain why it may be a possible cancer-preventive. Another effective technique explored under this heading is visualization therapy. This method has worked for many against varied conditions of ill health, including cancer. Finally, we report on a vitally important dietary supplement from Europe which scientists deservedly call a real breakthrough in the fight against cancer and other life-threatening conditions.

BE INFORMED

A WIDE VARIETY OF INFORMATION — This book is a serious effort to bring you information which may ease your mind by explaining the treatment your doctor judges best for medically treating an existing malignancy. Perhaps even more important is the material on the possible cancer-fighting nutritional and holistic methods you can put into practice yourself.

In this polluted world we live in, staying healthy is almost a full-time job. The knowledgeable, self-educated individual who takes the time to stay informed on the important advances in health care and preventive medicine has a better chance than most of enjoying good health into his sunset years.

The World of Science & Medicine
A Brief Review

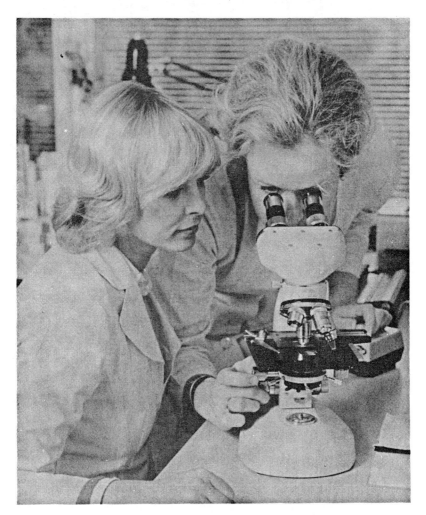

Chapter II

Is this the "Golden Age" of Cancer Research?

In the Footsteps of a Killer

If you believe everything you hear and read in the popular media, a cure for cancer is always just around the corner. Childhood cancer took a nosedive between 1973 and 1989. Death rates are down for some leukemias and cancers of the colon and rectum, stomach, uterus and cervix, bladder, skull, bone, gallbladder and testes.

Recent breakthroughs in human genetic engineering holds out hope that a cancer-linked DNA strand will soon be isolated and reprogrammed. Diagnostic improvements are catching more cancers in early treatable stages, so the disease is no longer an automatic death sentence.

But there's a dark side to all the hopefulness. John C. Bailar II, a professor of epidemiology and biostatistics at McGill University, has a history of raining on the cancer researchers' parades. In 1986, his formal study called "Progress Against Cancer?" caused a furious protest when it pointed out that the number of people facing cancer's bottom-line outcome - death - hadn't really changed much over the years.

Bailar stood before the President's Cancer Panel again in 1993. The news wasn't any better. More than 20 years and $25 billion after President Nixon declared war on the disease, the cancer mortality rate continues to rise, he said.

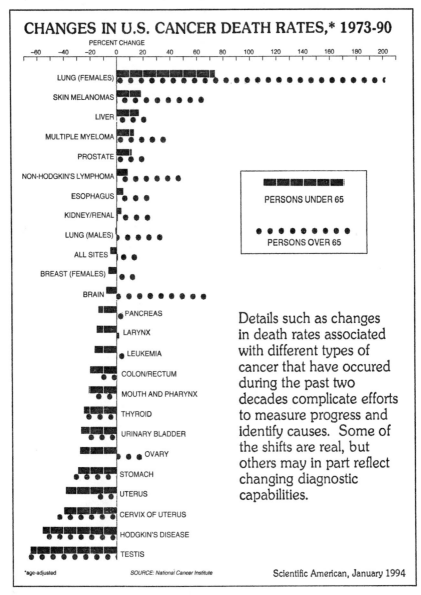

CHANGES IN U.S. CANCER DEATH RATES,* 1973-90

Details such as changes in death rates associated with different types of cancer that have occured during the past two decades complicate efforts to measure progress and identify causes. Some of the shifts are real, but others may in part reflect changing diagnostic capabilities.

*age-adjusted

SOURCE: National Cancer Institute

Scientific American, January 1994

"Any claim of major success against cancer must be reconciled to this figure," Bailar told the panel as he pointed to a graph of rising U.S. cancer death rates stretching from 1950 to 1990. "I do not think such reconciliation is possible. Again I conclude, as I did seven years ago, that our decades of war against cancer have been a qualified failure."

The National Cancer Institute estimates 526,000 cancer deaths occured in the United States in 1993. U.S. cancer death rates rose by 7 percent between 1975 and 1990. Cancer is still the second-leading cause of death in the country after heart disease.

U.S. Cancer Cases and Deaths in 1993*

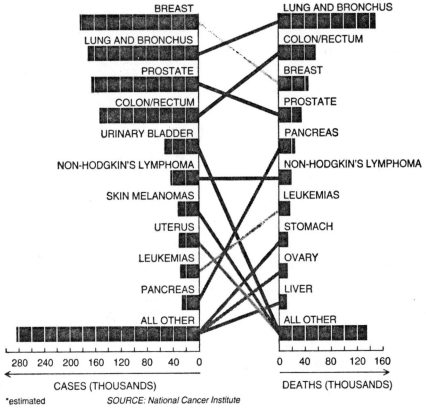

| 280 240 200 160 120 80 40 0 | 0 40 80 120 160 |
| CASES (THOUSANDS) | DEATHS (THOUSANDS) |

*estimated   SOURCE: National Cancer Institute

Scientific American, January 1994

Dr. Bailar and the Cancer Institute agree: most of these deaths are preventable. By far the greatest contributor to the increase was an explosion of lung cancer fatalities. Lung cancer, a disease suffered most frequently by cigarette smokers, causes almost a quarter of all cancer deaths. (Dr. Bailar considers these deaths "self-inflicted.") Lung cancer deaths increased almost 100 percent among women between 1973 and 1990. Melanoma and prostate cancers also displayed more than 80 percent increases during the same period.

Other cancers on the rise include those of the lymph nodes, brain, kidney, breast and esophagus. Even when lung cancer deaths are not considered by the statisticians, the total cancer death rate has changed little since the "war" started in 1971. Overall, the increases in cancer death rates - 18 percent - are twice as large as the decreases.

Relative Impact of Cancer in U.S. by Race, 1990

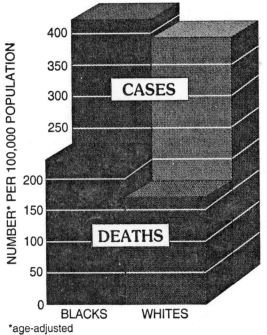

*age-adjusted

Source: Scientific American, January 1994

As the chart on page 23 shows, the prospects are even worse for African-Americans. For reasons that scientists can't explain, blacks in America who develop cancer die 35 percent more frequently than whites, even though the incidence of cancer among blacks is only 8 percent higher. Samuel Broder, head of the National Cancer Institute, said that a relative lack of access to health care might explain some of the discrepancy.

Another stumbling block to fighting the disease is the high cost of clinical trials. In order to meet strict Food and Drug Administration guidelines, any new treatment must be tried on thousands of volunteer patients over several years' time. The trials are usually run from major university hospitals, so many cancer patients have no access to the new technology.

Some researchers feel this is one reason cancer deaths among children have dropped. According to January 1994 article in *Scientific American* magazine, 80 percent of children with cancer enter experimental trials. Only 3 percent of adults do.

Politicians and scientists are re-thinking the agenda of the National Cancer Institute, wondering if all the money spent to find a cause and cure should instead go to prevention research.

What this means to you and me is that despite a worldwide crusade against it, our chances of surviving cancer today are not much better than they would have been thirty years ago - unless we take matters into our own hands. There are documented, effective preventive measures that can work to keep a body cancer-free for a lifetime. That is what this book is all about - ways to forestall cancer development before it begins, and treatments used to slow or stop cancer that is already established.

The NCI estimates that about a third of all cancers could be brought on by the patients' diet. Other scientists say that figure could go as high as 60 percent.

Strong evidence says that smoking and tobacco use is responsible for another third of all cancer deaths. Numbers of deaths linked to other causes aren't quite as clear-cut, but hard evidence exists to prove that alcohol, industrial chemicals, viruses and radiation also cause cells to turn malignant. Debate continues to rage over the cancer-causing effects of carcinogens in our air, food, water and workplaces.

Some of the theories and treatments outlined in this book espouse their own cancer causes, and many operate outside the accepted medical establishment. Although doctors are constrained to look askance at some of these theories, you, the consumer, must make the final decision about which treatment or prevention program is best for you.

A patient who thinks through each treatment with an open mind may outlive one who blindly follows the orders of his well-meaning physician. And one whose condition is terminal may finish out his days with less discomfort and indignity than those who buy a little more time by undergoing standard radiation and chemotherapy. A few even find their "terminal" cancers go into remission under these non-standard treatments, when all other hope is gone.

Another important factor is economic: with the price tag of some standard "last-ditch" cancer therapies reaching $100,000, those who opt for alternative therapies may still have something left to bequeath their children!

Those interested in more information on the President's Cancer Panel Meeting can obtain a free copy by mail by writing:

The National Cancer Institute
Department of Public Information
Bethesda, MD 20824

In the balance of this chapter, we're going to bring you up-to-date on the undeniably solid developments coming out of current scientific research. Here's what's going on.

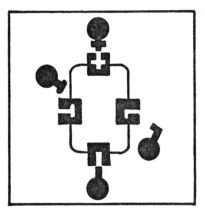

BIOLOGICAL MODIFIERS

Some new compounds attempt to convert cancer cells into normal ones. Others try to stimulate the body's immune system. And monoclonal antibodies, custom-made proteins similar to the body's natural defenders, may one day carry poisons directly to tumor cells.

BIOLOGICAL RESPONSE MODIFIERS — According to the National Cancer Institute, biological response modifiers appear very promising. The basic premise here is to stimulate (or restore) the body's own defenses so that all the potentially lethal anticancer forces of the body are mobilized and strengthened for the internal fight. All over the world, scientists are investigating ways to program the immune system to resist cancer and other diseases as well.

In the early 1980s, the NCI established BRMP (The Biological Response Modifiers Program) to identify and study new biological materials which fight cancer. Since that time, the BRMP researchers have identified hundreds of chemical substances which can influence the normal defenses of the body. Several groups of biological materials which are believed to be clinically important are currently being studied and tested.

THE IMMUNE SYSTEM — It is by producing antibodies and immune cells that the internal police system of the body fights disease. Antibodies, proteins which actively attack abnormal cells, and special white blood cells work within the immune system to surround and devour both diseased cells and viral invaders. *Macrophages* are the scavengers that gobble up foreign cells. The good news is that it has been determined that some chemical agents may be able to activate the macrophages, thereby stimulating the immune defense against malignant cells. Research is continuing.

INTERLEUKIN-2 — Steven Rosenberg, M.D. Ph.D., the Chief of Surgery at the NCI in Bethesda, Maryland has achieved what he himself cautiously calls a major breakthrough in man's continuing fight against cancer. Dr. Rosenberg says, "It's not a cancer cure in 1985, but it is a breakthrough in that it marks the first successful approach to using the body's own immune system to reject a cancer."

Interleukin-2 is a complex protein genetically programmed to boost the body's own white blood cells' ability to fight cancer. This space-age immunotherapy treatment involves hooking up the patient to cell-separating equipment which identifies and isolates a portion of the body's white blood cells. These disease-fighting cells, already a part of the vital immune system, are then mixed with interleukin-2 before they are returned to the bloodstream for their search and destroy mission.

The success of interleukin-2 is far from 100 percent. In the group of 25 patients accepted in the initial study, Dr. Rosenberg's NCI team reports that 11 patients had a 50 percent shrinkage in the size of their malignant tumors, but 14 patients did not respond and are still listed as terminal.

Although immunotherapy patients develop severe side effects, these effects are reversed at the close of the month-long treatment. Side effects include a weight-gain of up to 30 pounds because of fluid retention, which may lead to lung, kidney and liver disorders, plus flu-like symptoms such as chills, fever and diarrhea. Because patients accepted in the NCI program (only eight can be treated each month) are individuals who have not responded to conventional treatment and who are considered terminal, the side effects of interleukin-2 are risks most are eager to take.

Even though less than half of the patients involved in the clinical trials with interleukin-2 have responded favorably so far, medical science believes that further refinements of this immunotherapy program will increase the success rate considerably. Trials are continuing.

INTERFERON — Cancer research centers all over the globe, including six in the U.S., are studying interferon in clinical trials on human patients. The aim is to discover the maximum safe dosage, the quantity where maximum effect occurs, the best schedule of administration, and any possible toxic effects. In correlating the data, the NCI reports limited success and states that interferon is clearly beneficial in some respects.

A 50 percent reduction in tumor size has been documented in some few patients with breast cancer, melanoma, and other solid tumors. Results achieved in patients with kidney cancer were more promising and more than half of the leukemia patients involved responded favorably to interferon therapy. Side effects observed in patients include chills, fever, fatigue, decreased white blood cell count and abnormal liver function. However, when the interferon therapy was withdrawn, the side effects usually disappeared.

The theory here is that although interferon is not lethal to cancer, it apparently can slow malignant growth so that the cancerous cells no longer multiply and will eventually die. Laboratory studies with animals indicate that a combination of interferon and an anticancer drug may be more effective than using interferon alone. Research is proceeding on the theory that interferon will probably prove to be most useful in connection with other types of conventional cancer treatment.

AMPLIGEN — Ampligen, developed by scientists at John Hopkins University in Baltimore, is a highly promising biological response modifier. Because of its chemical formula, Ampligen is subject to enzymatic action in the blood and decomposes rapidly, but not before accomplishing its purpose. Because of this feature, Ampligen is less toxic than some of the other compounds under study as biological response modifiers. Ampligen also differs from some of the other drugs under investigation in that it doesn't stimulate the body's immune system to produce antibodies against it.

TUMOR NECROSIS FACTOR — TNF, or the tumor necrosis (killing) factor, is a substance (protein) produced naturally by *macrophages,* the white blood cells of the immune system that gobble up dangerous invaders. Tests in laboratory animals show that TNF acts directly on the defenses of the body by stimulating protective lymphocytes and macrophages. Researchers in both the U.S. and Japan have artificially produced TNF and trials in humans are scheduled, but the scientists agree it will be several years before TNF is approved for widespread use.

LIPOPHILIC MOLECULES — Lipophilic molecules bind with lipids (fats) in membranes. Researchers at the Dana-Farber Cancer Institute, affiliated with the prestigious Harvard Medical School (Cambridge, Massachusetts) have discovered that these charged compounds are released from normal cells, but remain active in carcinomas. Because carcinomas comprise 85 percent of human cancers, this is a very important finding.

Once a lipophilic molecule takes up residence in a cancer cell, it destroys the cell's ability to absorb enzymes necessary to its biochemical processes. These compounds have effectively inhibited the growth of human colon-carcinoma cells surgically implanted in laboratory mice. The lipophilic molecules currently being tested include *dequalinium* (an antibacterial agent), *rhodamine-123* (a dye used to change the color of laser light), and another compound used in industrial inks which has shown itself ten times more potent than dequalinium. The side effects observed in animals so far have been negligible.

HYDRAZINE — One of the truly awful effects of an advanced cancer is *cachexia,* a process of gradual starvation. Because a malignancy interferes with the normal metabolic process, the result is that the tumor absorbs the nutrients and the food consumed does not benefit the patient. Recent research indicates that in patients given hydrazine, an inexpensive and common industrial chemical, weight loss has been halted, even though their cancers were well advanced. The American Cancer Society has ordered a two-year study, now commencing its second year, on the action of hydrazine in patients with colorectal cancers.

LIGHT TREATMENT — Speaking at the American Cancer Society seminar in mid-1985, Dr. Richard Edelson of Columbia University described his process for treating blood outside the body with a drug (psoralen) which is activated by ultraviolet light. Edelson's light treatment, called *extracorporeal photophoresis* (extra [outside] corporeal [physical body] photo [Greek 'light'] phoresis [the migration of charged ions through a membrane]), involves injecting the patient with psoralen which is known to attack defective immune cells. Because psoralen is activated only by untraviolet light, two hours after administration of the drug, a portion of the patient's blood supply is removed and the white blood cells are isolated. The psoralen-saturated white blood cells are then exposed to ultraviolet radiation for less than a second and the activated blood is returned to the patient.

The Columbia University group has treated 11 patients suffering from a particularly deadly form of cancer (cutaneous T cell lymphoma) which allows its victims an average survival time of only three to five years. Two of the 11 patients have been able to discontinue treatment and remain free of cancer. Eight have shown a marked decrease in the lethal T cells.

Edelson cautions that extracorporeal photophoresis is not a cure, explaining that it eliminates some of the T cells, but doesn't stop the body from producing them altogether. Edelson says, "What we are really after is the treatment of immune diseases. I think the future for immunotherapy is very bright. In combination with other therapies, this approach may lead to good control of cancer."

In autoimmune diseases, the immune system itself goes off track and attacks the body. It is speculated that Edelson's combination drug and light therapy may also prove useful in the treatment of rheumatoid arthritis and lupus.

LASERS — In a process called *photodynamic therapy*, scientists are using an innovative combination of drugs and the laser beam to destroy cancerous growths. A non-toxic drug is administered which sensitizes cancerous lesions to light. After three days, a laser beam is directed on the tumor for 8 to 10 minutes.

The Roswell Park Memorial Institute (Buffalo, New York) has reported preliminary testing of over 3,000 cancer patients suffering with lung or bladder cancer treated by this new therapy has given some encouraging results. Between 25 to 35 percent of the patients in this study were tumor-free thirty days after treatment.

HYPERTHERMIA — A modified food-warming oven consisting of a chamber that produces radiant heat up to 108 degrees Fahrenheit appears to enhance the benefits of chemotherapy and radiation without adding further toxic side effects.

Trials conducted at the University of Wisconsin Medical School by H. Ian Robins used heat therapy on cancer patients suffering from a number of different forms of cancer. In this procedure, Dr. Robins brought the body temperature of his patients up to 107.4 degrees F. and maintained temperature for up to three hours. He reports four patients with lymphoma had a favorable response to a combination of radiation therapy and the hyperthermia technique.

Dr. Robins explains, "The advantage of whole-body hyperthermia is that it gets at disseminated cancer and boosts the beneficial effects of both chemotherapy and radiation."

CANCER-SPECIFIC AGENTS

MONOCLONAL ANTIBODIES — Monoclonal antibodies (MABs) are artificial antibodies laboratory produced to search out and destroy specific cancers. An important feature of MABs is that their destructive effect can be increased by impregnating them with a powerful anticancer drug before injecting them into the body. Because the lethal anticancer drugs currently used in chemotherapy are not cancer-specific but also destroy normal cells, this particular line of scientific endeavor may prove to be the most exciting yet.

The Scripps Clinic & Research Foundation in La Jolla, California has used MABs successfully against human tumors which were established by transplantation into lab mice. A patient in his mid-60s suffering from lymph cancer was treated at Stanford University with MABs. The treatment completely destroyed the malignancy. Children with leukemia given MAB therapy at the Dana Farber Cancer Institute have also benefited.

The most comprehensive study of MAB therapy comes from Dr. Hilary Koprowski, Director of the Wistar Institute of Anatomy & Biology in Philadelphia. Dr. Koprowski has

31

revealed results of a study of 50 cancer victims given monoclonal antibodies after they had failed to benefit from conventional treatment. Follow-ups from two to four years after the MAB therapy showed that two patients were free of any malignancy; in ten patients, the normal progress of the disease was permanently slowed; and in 25 other victims, there was at least a temporary beneficial response.

MABs may also prove to be an extremely valuable diagnostic tool. A cancer-specific MAB impregnated with a radioactive substance and then given intravenously will travel to minute cancer cells wherever they are located within the body. By scanning with special equipment, cancer can be detected by this method before conventional diagnostic methods are able to distinguish any tiny malignancy.

IMMUNOTOXINS — The production of a safe cancer-specific immunotoxin is accomplished by injecting cancer cells into a laboratory mouse. The mouse's immune system then produces antibodies having the ability to bind with the antigen site on the cancer cells. A toxin (which may be bacterial, botanical, or chemical) is added. This produces an immunotoxin antibody with the ability to bind to the antigen on the cancer cell and destroy it. The cancer-specific immunotoxin cannot bind with the antigen site of normal cells and they are bypassed.

Although the concept appears simple and laboratory tests are promising, a number of questions must be answered before doctors are willing to risk injecting an immunotoxin directly into the body. The immunotoxin must be safe for normal tissue, stable within the body's very complex environment, and cancer-specific.

To avoid any potentially unknown destructive complications, Dr. Daniel Vallera, University of Minnesota Medical School, is studying the effect of treating bone marrow cells outside the body with immunotoxins. Conventional treatment of patients with bone cancer and leukemia often includes chemotherapy and whole-body radiation treatment, which destroys normal cells in the bone marrow which are the vital precursors of all blood cells. By using immunotoxins outside the body, Vallera demonstrated their effectiveness with minimum destruction of normal cells. The benefits of treating bone marrow in this way are now being cautiously tested on patients.

Experiments injecting immunotoxins directly into the bloodstream of a guinea pig with liver cancer conducted by Michael Bernhard of the NCI and his associates met with limited success. The group reported that a single injection shrank the tumor, but did not completely destroy it.

The hope is that a number of immunotoxins can be developed with each specific against the different types of cancer cells, but safe for normal cells. Many researchers are working on doing just that.

CANCER VACCINES — Results from an on-going study begun in 1981 by Michael G. Hanna and H. C. Hoover under the auspices of Litton Bionetics, Inc., Rockville, Maryland, indicate that a cancer vaccine might soon be a reality. Twenty cancer patients were given injections of their own malignant cells after colorectal tumor surgery. The cancer cells were first treated with radiation so that they could not reproduce and a total of three vaccinations, the first two combined with an immune system enhancer, were given each patient.

All twenty of the vaccinated patients experienced good results. None has died and only four suffered a recurrence of cancer. On the other hand, twenty colorectal cancer patients operated on at approximately the same time, but not given the vaccine, did not fare so well. Four have died of cancer and another five have recurring malignancies.

At the Roswell Park Memorial Institute in Buffalo, Heinz Kohler is working to develop an anti-idiotype vaccine which he believes will destroy the body's tolerance to a tumor. Kohler explains, "The immune system identifies shapes, but doesn't care what's behind those shapes. The idiotype provides an antibody that could be a substitute for the original antigen."

Dr. Kohler estimates that human studies are at least two or three years away, but hopes to have a vaccine ready to begin animal trials by the middle of 1986.

CONTROLLING METASTASIS — Finding a way to keep a

cancer localized and prevent *metastasis* (spreading) to another area of the body is a dream of oncologists all over the world. Researchers at the Georgetown University School of Medicine (Washington, D.C.) believe they have taken an important first step in doing just that. They appear to have discovered the way in which malignant cells escape a localized tumor and travel to another site.

A protein called *fibronectin* is a part of what holds both normal cells and cancerous cells together. When the connecting fibronectin breaks down in a cancerous cell, the malignant cell is freed and enters the bloodstream or lymphatic system where it can migrate throughout the body. Using chicken embryo cells infected with RSV (Rous sarcoma virus), which causes a cancer of the connective tissue in chickens, the scientists determined that a viral enzyme (*pp60src*, a product of RSV's cancer-causing gene), degraded the fibronectin holding the cancer cells together and allowed them to float free. The researchers concluded that without the viral enzyme, the fibronectin would remain intact. With its fibronectin intact, a cancer cell would be held in place and could not metastasize elsewhere in the body.

AS THINGS STAND NOW

It's all very good and well to look forward to a future when a 'magic bullet' containing a cancer-specific agent may possibly be developed which will kill and destroy a malignancy without harming normal tissue. In the meantime, the medical community must fight cancer with the limited means at their command. The following chapter describes the medical approach to the treatment of cancer as things stand now.

Chapter III

Orthodox Medical Treatment

Surgery, Radiation, & Chemotherapy

As science works overtime attempting to discover less damaging treatments, procedures, and chemical drugs which are cancer-specific and not toxic to normal cell tissue, medical oncologists and surgeons are fighting back with the only weapons in their arsenal.

According to the U.S. Department of Health & Human Services, 20 percent of those diagnosed as having cancer are in a stage too far advanced to be termed 'curable.' In the remaining 80 percent (those who stand a chance of a complete cure or permanent remission of the disease), surgery is the treatment of choice in 45 percent. In an additional 10 percent, surgery combined with radiation therapy is the primary method of attack.

Radiation alone is given in approximately 20 percent of the cases diagnosed. Less than 10 percent of those suffering from cancer receive chemotherapy as their first form of treatment. However, chemotherapy is considered useful for the large number of cancer victims who suffer a recurrence of some form of this dread disease.

EARLY WARNING SYSTEM

The entire health-care industry is now engaged in some important changes in the way both primary (preventive) measures and secondary (screening) controls against cancer are being handled. A massive preventive campaign has been launched by the National Cancer Institute in order to reduce the incidence of cancer cases by the year 2000.

There's been a spurt of growth in the number of health maintenance organizations (HMOs) recently and many hospitals have expanded their outpatient facilities as well. It's easier now than it's ever been to catch cancer in its early stages. The experts say that early detection is the key to a complete cure.

In an address before the American Society of Preventive Oncology (April, 1985), Sam Shapiro, B.S., of the Health Services Research & Development Center (Baltimore, Maryland) showed the importance of detecting a malignancy in its earliest form by explaining the progress against three different cancers (breast, cervix, colorectal).

Breast Cancer — Under the auspices of the National Cancer Institute, the Health Insurance Plan (HIP) initiated a study of the efficacy of routinely scanning the breast for cancer back in the early 1960s. The subjects in the study were subjected to a physical examination of the breast and three additional exams, including mammography, each year for the period of the study (early 1960s to early 1970s). What the ten-year long HIP study showed was that clinical examination of the breast, coupled with routine mammography, can reduce the projected death rate of breast cancer by up to 30 percent.

A later study, dubbed the Breast Cancer Detection Demonstration Project (BCDDP), included a wide sample of women (250,000) aged 35 to 74 years. This nationwide study was implemented in 1973, again under the sponsorship of the NCI. A total of twenty-seven cancer screening centers were required to complete the full cycle of five annual screenings using physical palpitation and examination of the breast, plus mammography, and thermography on each of the women.

Because of the justifiable concern over subjecting the women to high radiation exposure during screening, every effort was made to reduce exposure to the absolute minimum. One important advancement came out of this study. The scientists determined that it was possible to reduce the radiation dose to the breast midline well below 1 rad per exam without reducing the effectiveness of the screening. Thanks to these improved screening procedures, more and more patients and physicians alike are welcoming this method of detecting a small malignancy which is easy to surgically remove.

However, the experts say that methods for preventing the occurrence of breast cancer are far from clear while emphasizing the absolute necessity of early detection. Many of us are paying attention. A 1979 survey of women aged 20 to 64 years of age revealed that 63 percent had had a breast examination by a doctor within the past year, and another 20 percent said they had had such an examination within the past two years. By far, most women said that their physician had suggested the examination. One negative finding came out of this survey, however. Only one woman out of five reported having had a mammogram.

Cervical Cancer — Although the effectiveness of the Pap test has been questioned for a number of years, health specialists agree that this is a useful early detection procedure against cancer of the cervix. Most physicians routinely take a Pap smear during a physical examination. In other words, if you're a woman and go to the doctor for just about any reason, one of the questions you can expect is, "How long has it been since you had a Pap test?"

Surveys show that more than 70 percent of the women tallied had a Pap smear test regularly. Of this 70 percent, close to 60 percent reported having had a Pap test during the twelve months prior to the survey and another 20 percent reported having had the test within twenty-four months of the survey.

Overall, the death rate from cervical cancer has gone down slightly in recent years, but it can't be classified as a low risk. Especially at risk are the economically disadvantaged groups not covered by health care plans. For these people, routine physical examinations which include a Pap smear test (and breast examination) are not a reality of life. Without early detection, cancer of the cervix still kills.

Colorectal Cancer — For the population as a whole, the early detection of cancer of the colon or rectum just doesn't happen. Not enough doctors employ the use of the proctoscope to peer into the rectum, and few patients want to undergo this unpopular procedure. However, it must be pointed out that oncologists (cancer specialists) uniformly agree that a proctoscopic examination is the surest way to detect the early development of colorectal cancers. The experts say that once proctoscopy becomes a routine part of a general physical exam, we can look for a substantial reduction in the death rate of this type of cancer.

DO YOUR PART

Detecting a mass of cancerous (or precancerous) cells in its earliest stage gives you the best chance to beat it. Cancers which have not progressed to the stage where they produce noticeable symptoms are usually small, localized, and easily removed.

The American Cancer Society says that all of us should be intimately familiar with our bodies. Women are directed to examine their breasts monthly and be on the alert for lumps, a new thickening in the tissue, or any other change. Men are advised to be aware of the normal size and consistency of their testicles and to check them monthly for any change in the contour, an enlargement, or a difference in the degree of hardness.

The *Seven Warning Signals* of cancer are probably familiar to most of us, but they bear repeating. Watch out for:
1. Unusual bleeding or discharge
2. A lump or thickening (breast or elsewhere)
3. A sore that does not heal
4. A change in bowel or bladder habits
5. A persistent cough or hoarseness
6. Difficulty in swallowing or continual indigestion
7. A change in a wart or mole

Although the occurrence of any of these symptoms does not

necessarily mean you have cancer, the American Cancer Society recommends that you see your doctor immediately if any of these warning signals lasts longer than two weeks.

REGULAR PHYSICAL EXAM — A regular and thorough physical examination can be very useful in detecting even an early and symptomless malignancy. Your physican should conduct a detailed visual examination and palpitation of your entire body. His trained eyes and hands can spot an abnormality that might escape your notice. He will pay special attention to all body cavities, including the mouth, vagina, bladder (urogenital area), and rectum.

For some reason, all of us seem to reject the idea of a *proctosigmoidoscopy,* the examination of the rectum with a lighted tube. This simple and painless ten-minute procedure, albeit a little undignified, is extremely important in the early detection (and cure) of *colorectal* cancer, a malignant tumor of the colon or rectum. This type of examination is especially important for males because it will often show any prostate involvement as well.

Statistics show that the current death rate of women suffering from cervical cancer could be reduced by up to 90 percent if a yearly vaginal smear test (PAP) was a part of a regular physical examination. All women over 50 years of age are advised to have a soft-tissue x-ray (mammogram) of the breasts as well. Authorities say that, beginning at age 30, young women with a family history of breast cancer should have a baseline mammogram at least every other year.

ADDITIONAL DIAGNOSTIC PROCEDURES — *X-rays,* including the newer *CAT* scan (computer-aided tomography) which provides a more detailed visualization of internal masses than the original type of x-rays, give the physician a peek at what's going on internally. *Ultrasound,* high-frequency sound waves, registers differences in tissue and organ density and can show any abnormal changes which might be occurring.

A wide variety of *biochemical laboratory tests* on urine and blood can be useful in detecting specific cancers and are also used to monitor the effectiveness of treatment. *Cytology,* the microscopic examination of cell smears (taken from the mucous membranes of the nose, mouth, stomach and saliva) is a common early diagnostic procedure, but the results are considered inconclusive.

Most physicians prefer to follow up with an actual *biopsy* before diagnosing cancer. In a biopsy, a small piece of suspect tissue is surgically removed, stained, and viewed under a microscope for any tell-tale abnormalities. When indications of a possible cancer are strong, very often an anesthetized patient is kept on the table in the operating room while the tissue is being examined. This allows the physician to surgically remove the mass if laboratory tests confirm the presence of malignancy.

A *pathological* diagnosis of cancer is dependent on both the appearance of the biopsied tissue sample under a high-powered electron microscope and the clinical outcome of the case. In this type of procedure, the biochemical characteristics of the cells are critical and must be precisely evaluated by an expert laboratory pathologist.

In most instances, the management of a cancer patient's care and treatment is handled by an expert group of specialists, including a medical oncologist, surgeon, radiotherapist, and pathologist. These authorities consult with one another and minutely examine the details of the case to determine the best way to proceed.

TREATMENT: A LIMITED ARSENAL

SURGERY — The most effective way to eliminate cancer is to simply remove it surgically, along with neighboring tissue which may be suspect. When surgery is used in combination with advanced techniques employing radiation and chemotherapy, medical science has found that it is not really necessary to amputate an entire limb or breast to eradicate the cancer. The medical procedures available to the cancer specialist today have vastly improved in just the past five years alone.

In fact, you might want to spare a moment or two to be thankful that you are living in the modern world. It was not until the 19th century, when anesthesia and the benefit of antiseptic conditions were discovered, that surgery became a relatively safe and viable option for patients of the day. Further medical advances in the 20th century included immense improvements in surgical techniques, the introduction of blood transfusions, and powerful antibiotics to control infection.

Today, heart-lung pumps, artificial kidneys, the replacement of bones and blood vessels, plus the transplant of entire organs, seem almost commonplace. With these important further advances, suddenly all parts of the body have become accessible to the surgeon's knife.

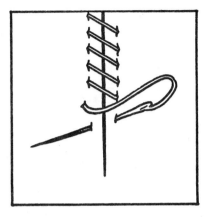

SURGERY
Surgery to remove a tumor and nearby tissue remains the most effective way to cure many cancers. With radiation and chemotherapy, fewer amputations of limbs and breasts are performed than once were.

Although even more scientific and medical advances are coming slowly, surgically removing (excising) a cancerous mass completely is currently considered the optimum method of eliminating a malignancy. And it is, provided the tumor is enclosed and has not metastasized (spread) to other areas of the body.

From the time of Hippocrates, the abiding principle of medicine has always been *primum non nocere,* meaning "first, do no harm." Any surgeon worth his salt knows that there is an additional risk involved in 'opening up' any patient, particularly a cancer victim. If it is impossible to completely remove the malignancy, surgery can speed up the spread of cancer cells and actually shorten the life of the patient.

However, even when it is known in advance that a widespread cancer involving vital organs cannot be completely cut out, a surgeon can relieve the agonizing pain that is characteristic of some malignancies by severing critical nerve pathways. In addition, surgery may be necessary to relieve an internal obstruction or remove an abscess arising from either infection or the tumor itself.

As a valuable preventive measure, the physician may advise surgical removal of precancerous polyps in the colon or rectum, nodules in the thyroid gland, the uterus, certain pigmented moles, chronic ulcers, and some precancerous conditions arising inside the mouth.

Twenty years ago, a woman with a suspect lump in her breast often went into the operating room without knowing for certain whether she would undergo a complete *mastectomy* (surgical removal of the breast and neighboring nerves, muscles, lymph nodes, and tissue). If the waiting pathologist determined that her biopsied tissue was cancerous, the surgeon completely cut away the breast in an honest attempt to insure that all malignancy was eliminated.

Today, many women are considered candidates for a less disfiguring *lumpectomy,* in which merely the cancerous tumor and a small amount of surrounding tissue is removed. The good news is that a recent federally funded study of 1,843 breast-cancer patients shows that the five-year survival rate was 85 percent for women undergoing a lumpectomy in contrast to a 76 percent survival rate for women who had the complete mastectomy. In lumpectomy patients who were subsequently given radiation treatment, only 7.7 percent developed a recurring tumor in the same breast as opposed to 27.9 percent of those who had the lumpectomy only.

Women who must undergo a complete mastectomy because of extensive involvement will be glad to learn that breast reconstruction is becoming more and more common. The surgeon can save the nipple and sufficient skin, insert a prosthesis to match the natural breast, and then re-position the nipple in its normal place. Because the nerves have been cut, the nipple will no longer be sensitive to touch, but the appearance of the reconstructed breast is completely natural.

RADIATION THERAPY — In 1895, Wilhelm Roentgen discovered that electromagnetic rays had a rare power to penetrate animal tissue and give a picture of the internal workings of the body. Dubbed x-rays, this procedure was immediately acclaimed as an important diagnostic aid. It was not until 1910 that science determined that x-rays could lead to the development of cancer. But, on the other hand, skin cancers exposed to x-rays (or radium) disappeared. Now we come to the heart of the problem; how much exposure is valuable (and an acceptable risk in continuing to use x-rays in diagnosis and treatment) and how much is too much?

Radiotherapy treatment uses a source of ionizing radiation, such as x-rays, radium, or radioactive cobalt, for the destruction of malignant cancer cells. The trick is to bombard the complete cancerous mass (and any extensions or offshoots) with radiation at the precise application which will destroy the tumor, but only cause minimal damage to normal tissue. The aim is to allow normal tissue to recover and survive the bombardment.

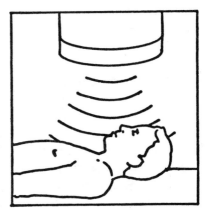

RADIATION THERAPY
Computerized controls, better methods of pinpointing the tumor, and new forms of radiation allow more selective destruction of tumors while sparing normal tissue. Chemicals are being tested to heighten a cancer's sensitivity to radiation.

With the development of multimillion volt equipment, high-speed delivery accomplishes a deeper and more sure penetration of tissue, more precise and sharper delineation of the field under attack, and less involvement of the neighboring normal tissue. Even newer types of sub-atomic particles (protons, neutrons, helium ions, pions) are being investigated for possible ways with which to increase the beneficial effects and broaden the range of this type of treatment.

43

Certain tumors (of the pancreas, stomach, esophagus, head, neck) have a strong resistance to conventional radiation therapy and some cancers are judged inoperable because they have invaded vital organs. It is these types of malignancies that science hopes will prove vulnerable to the more versatile forms of radiation. The results are encouraging and many researchers are expressing a guarded optimism.

Radiation is commonly used before a scheduled surgery to shrink the tumor to a more operable size. A new procedure, tested on more than 400 patients at U.S. cancer centers, involves bombarding the tumor directly with a massive dose of radiation during surgery while the patient is on the operating table. By directly targeting the area, there is no covering tissue in the way to sustain damage and very little involvement of neighboring tissue. The NCI cautions that it's too soon to evaluate long-term results in comparison with orthodox radiation therapy.

The aim of the radiologist is always to protect normal tissue while delivering a lethal dose of radiation to every malignant cell in a cancerous tumor. Another method of direct delivery being tested is the implant of a radioactive pellet into the tumor itself. Several types of malignancies, including breast cancer and prostatic cancer, are possible candidates for this type of treatment. The dose of radiation delivered to the tumor is maximized, while little can spill over into normal tissue.

NEUTRONS — According to data coming from the University of Washington (Seattle, Washington), neutrons (non-electric sub-atomic particles) have been used in the treatment of over 6000 patients, both here in the U.S. and abroad. Statistics appear to indicate that neutron radiation offers a strong advantage in the management of salivary gland tumors and prostatic cancer, but a only a slight advantage against bone, cartilege, and soft tissue malignancies.

PIONS — Pions or pi mesons (electrically charged particles of mass sized midway between electrons and protons) are being used in extensive medical trials at the Los Alamos National Laboratory (New Mexico). In 20 male patients suffering from prostatic cancer treated solely with pions, local control was achieved in 18. However, these very encouraging results were offset by the fact that only two patients out of a total of 59 victims of brain tumors (malignant glioma) responded favorably to pion irradiation.

Medical scientists in Switzerland experimenting with pion treatment report that this method has an excellent future against bladder cancer. In a group of 55 bladder cancer patients, the Swiss claim a complete response in 19 with total local control of the malignancy.

PROTONS — The Harvard Cyclotron Laboratory (Cambridge, Massachusetts) currently supplies four different hospitals and health-care facilities with protons (charged atomic particles) for their respective cancer treatment centers. Over the past decade, 965 patients have been irradiated with proton beams. Almost 600 of this group were being treated for a cancer in the back of the eyeball (choroidal melanoma), notoriously difficult to eliminate or control without complete removal of the eyeball itself. The proton treatment chalked up an astounding local control rate of 98 percent.

In a group of 67 patients with a rare form of cancer (chordoma or chondrosarcoma: tumor formed at the base of the skull or spine), the local control rate was a very satisfactory 89 percent of those treated with proton beams. This figure was confirmed and locked in more than a year after treatment during a follow-up evaluation of each patient.

Unfortunately, those being treated with protons for an inoperable brain tumor (glioma) did not fare so well. Of the seven patients thus treated, only one can be considered a long-term survivor. The other six died within a few months of completing treatment.

HELIUM IONS — The University of California (San Francisco, California) has also reported success against spinal cord tumors (chondrosarcomas) and eye tumors (choroidal melanonomas). Using helium ions (a combination of two protons and two neutons), these medical scientists have treated 190 patients suffering with a tumor behind the eyeball and report achieving local control in 116. A total of 27 of the group developed cataracts, making cataracts a significant complication of treatment. Inasmuch as cataract surgery is routinely performed today, that would seem to be a fair tradeoff.

Although the California researchers have treated only 19 patients with cancerous spinal cord involvement, local control was achieved in 15. Control has been documented in follow-up evaluations ranging from two months to over two years in some of the cases.

Working against time, as did the physicians of previous centuries, the radiologists of our time are now involved in an intensive evaluation of the different sources of ionizing radiation and are attempting to work out the filtration, distance factors, and sequence of doses best used against the wide variety of cancers that respond poorly to conventional radiation and other forms of treatment.

CHEMOTHERAPY — At its most optimistic and hopeful, *chemotherapy* is defined as "the application of chemical reagents which are not harmful to the patient, but which have a specific and toxic effect on disease-causing micro-organisms." (Taber's Cyclopedic Medical Dictionary). Unfortunately, we've all heard horror stories of the debilitating and sometimes agonizing side-effects of chemotherapy.

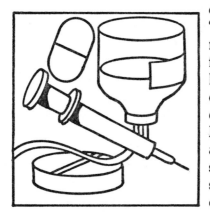

CHEMOTHERAPY
Scientists are working to limit the side effects of chemotherapy. Some are searching for new toxic agents to kill cancer cells, while others are synthesizing less toxic cousins of existing drugs. Combinations of drugs have proved more effective than single-drug treatments.

However, this is not to imply that chemotherapy is a treatment to be avoided at all costs. Certain cancers respond very favorably to this treatment, including *choriocarcinoma* (tumor originating in the placenta), and *Burkitt's lymphoma* (tumor of the lymph system). The cure rate of chemotherapy against these two particularly malignant forms of cancer is very high. Children suffering from acute *leukemia* (blood cancer) treated with a combination of chemotherapy drugs often enjoy long-term periods of disease-free remission, as do patients in even the most advanced stages of *Hodgkin's disease,* which affects the spleen, liver, and lymphoid tissue.

In an attempt to overcome one of the most debilitating effects of some chemotherapy drugs, scientists are testing new anti-nausea agents to prevent the uncontrolled vomiting and severe nausea that causes some patients to refuse treatment. Showing great promise as a nausea preventive is *nabilone,* one of the effective ingredients in marijuana. When nabilone is given before chemotherapy begins, nausea can be reduced to bearable proportions.

One of the problems faced by medical science is the fact that most cancer drugs have a limited usefulness. In a tumor, only a certain percentage of the malignant cells are dividing at any given time. Most drugs can effectively destroy only the part of the cells undergoing division. Some cancer cells develop a resistance to the drugs and render them ineffective. An even greater problem is the fact that tumor cells require such a large amount of a drug to destroy them that normal cells are destroyed as well.

In order to overcome these effects, combinations of chemo-therapeutic agents which act on cells in different ways are used in various treatment programs, either simultaneously or in a measured sequence. By combining or varying the drugs used, there is less irreparable damage to normal cells and the tendency of malignant cells to become resistant to a single agent is counteracted.

COMBINING DRUGS — The National Cancer Institute reports that encouraging results are attained with the combination of *adriamycin,* a common anticancer chemotherapeutic agent, and *verapamil.* Verapamil is a drug used to control heart *arrhythmias* (irregular heartbeat). NCI researchers say that the evidence gathered thus far indicates that the addition of verapamil can counter the ability of some cancer cells to resist chemotherapy.

Although it is known to destroy kidney cells, *cisplatin* is nevertheless a valuable and widely used chemotherapy drug. Scientists have determined that when the patient is infused with a saline (salt) solution along with cisplatin, the salt renders the cisplatin less toxic to kidney cells, giving the drug time to attack the cancer.

The cisplatin/saline combination proved beneficial in women with ovarian cancer and men with third-stage (advanced) cancer of the testicles. With a projected cure rate of only 50 percent by the usual treatment, the cure rate of men given this combination therapy jumped to a very encouraging 85 to 90 percent.

However, given the protective effect exerted on the kidney cells by the saline solution, another problem surfaced. Cisplatin is also highly toxic to nerve cells. The NCI is now working to find a way to counteract this additional barrier to the use of cisplatin.

CIRCADIAN TIMING — Another factor under study is the circadian timing of drug administration. In dissecting this term, we find *circa* (about) *dian* (day) refers to the fact that certain biological rhythms of the body are known to occur approximately every 24 hours. Studies have shown that simply taking these internal biological changes into account and timing the administration of adriamycin and cisplatin accordingly has a profound effect on the body's ability to handle the toxicity of the drugs.

A paper issued by the University of Minnesota Medical School and the Masonic Cancer Center (Minneapolis, Minnesota) says that "The most crucial element in the successful application of cancer chemotherapy is optimization of the effects and minimization of toxicity to normal tissue. One approach to increasing this selectivity is administration of these highly toxic drugs at times associated with best tolerance."

In a study of the effects of cherotherapy on 31 patients suffering with advanced ovarian cancer, the researchers found that the administration of *adriamycin in the morning* and *cisplatin in the evening* was more easily tolerated and resulted in far fewer side effects and consequent interruption of treatment. For instance, in the control group receiving the drugs in the reverse order, drug dosages had to be modified downward three times as often, complications and side effects were doubled, and four times as many treatments had to be delayed while the patient regained the strength to continue.

DRUGS DISGUISED — In another attempt to lessen the toxicity of chemotherapy agents to normal cell tissue, both the University of North Carolina Medical School (Chapel Hill, North Carolina) and the University of Illinois (Urbana, Illinois) have bound anticancer drugs, such as adriamycin, to the same type of protein that is found in a common blood clot. A drug in the guise of a blood clot doesn't bind as easily to normal cells. Cells in the area of a malignant tumor gobble up the protein, therby releasing the drug and activating it directly at the site of the cancer.

A spokesman for the University of North Carolina explains, "For most anticancer drugs, the difference between the toxic dose and the effective dose is pitifully small. By taking advantage of the biochemical differences between normal and malignant cells, we don't necessarily make the drugs more effective for fighting cancer, just less toxic to normal cells."

CANCER CONTROL

Preventing cancer from invading your body is the best defense, but controlling cancer by finding it early is an important and viable second line of defense available to us all. The National Cancer Institute is going all out on a strong program of education and is encouraging state health agencies and industry to implement their own risk assessment programs. Health maintenance organizations are springing up everywhere. At the end of 1985, over 400 HMOs with a combined membership of close to 20 million were functioning. For these 20 million people, regular physical examinations utilizing advanced cancer detection procedures are a reality. Efficient screening programs have been shown to be invaluable in the control of cancer.

IS THE KILLER WINNING? — As things stand right now, we appear to be willing to settle for a draw. Even with all its considerable forces mobilized and on the attack, medical science cannot say just when cancer will be conquered. To be sure, we are taking two giant steps forward in the fight against cancer for every one step backward. We are inching toward a better understanding of the various forms of the disease and trying new and more effective methods of treatment and therapy every year. The most brilliant scientific and medical minds in the world are working to find a solution to this condition which frightens even the most fearless among us, *but . . .*

PREVENTION REMAINS THE BEST SOLUTION — There are many natural and holistic ways with which you can help yourself. You must examine your lifestyle and make whatever changes necessary in order to protect yourself and your loved ones from the spectre stalking us all. You can be a victor and not a victim. We can point the way, but only you can make the right choices.

Chapter IV

Diet as a Weapon

Cancer is a fearful disease because terminal patients die so slowly and painfully. Cancer is the second most common cause of death in America - just behind heart disease. Cancer effects one of every three Americans. Nutrition, lifestyle and everyday environments create the most common cancer risks. These risks can be reduced by dietary and lifestyle changes.

The National Cancer Institute acknowledges the role of diet on cancer. Since 1992, it has recommended Americans eat five daily servings of both fruits and vegetables as part of a low-fat, high-fiber diet.

Dietary problems faced by United States citizens, published by the Senate Select Committee on Nutrition and Human Needs, looks like this:

1. Americans eat too much

2. Americans eat too much meat and fat

3. Americans eat too much sugar

4. Americans eat too much salt

5. Americans' diets lack fruits, vegetables and grains

6. Americans' diets are comprised of up to 45 percent fats

Healthy fat intake is 30 percent or less of the total day's intake.

Research published by the Cancer Institute supports the link between diet and cancer control. It found:

1. Diet and nutrition are factors in 60 percent of cancers in women
2. Diet and nutrition are factors in 40 percent of cancers in men
3. Nutrition is closely related to the formation or prevention of gastrointestinal cancers (stomach, pancreas and esophagus); breast cancer; prostate cancer; endometrial cancer

With knowledge comes hope: We have some control over the risk factors. Through diet we can fight cancer, the nation's number-two killer.

Later in this volume I will detail the FDA's new "Food Pyramid," a basic guide to daily nutrition. (See chapter 13). For now, I will concentrate on cancer-specific foods and dietary advice.

DIETARY RECOMMENDATIONS FROM THE NATIONAL CANCER INSTITUTE

The National Cancer Institute and nutritionists at the federal Food and Drug Administration agree that Americans should eat more fiber and reduce their fat intake. Freshness counts - both authorities stress nutrition lost when fruits and vegetables are cooked and processed. Calcium is also important, they say - a lifetime of low calcium intake can lead to osteoporosis, a brittle bone disease that strikes the elderly - mostly women.

The American Health Academy recommends Americans under age 25 take at least 1200 milligrams of calcium each day. After age 40, the dosage should increase to 1500 mg. per day. To create strong bones without adding fat to your diet, simply integrate non-fat milk and dairy products into your daily menu.

Milk isn't the only source of calcium. The June 1993 issue of *Prevention* magazine focused on calcium. It recommends taking a calcium supplement as well as daily servings of the foods listed below.

CALCIUM FOODS THAT CARRY THE MOST CLOUT

1 cup plain nonfat yogurt	400 mg per serving
1 cup nonfat milk	300 mg per serving
1 cup fruit nonfat yogurt	350 mg per serving
1 cup calcium-fortified orange juice	300 mg per serving
1 oz. nonfat cheese	200 mg per serving
1 cup "Calcimilk"	500 mg per serving

(lactose-reduced, calcium added.)

FDA CONSUMER JOURNAL'S TOP 20 FRUITS, VEGETABLES AND FISH

TOP 20 FRUITS	VEGETABLES	FISH
Banana	potato	shrimp
apple	lettuce	cod
watermelon	tomato	pollock
orange	onion	catfish
cantaloupe	carrot	scallop
grape	celery	salmon
grapefruit	sweet corn	flounder
strawberry	broccoli	sole
peach	green cabbage	oyster
pear	cucumber	orange roughy
nectarine	bell pepper	mackerel
honeydew melon	cauliflower	ocean perch
plum	leaf lettuce	rockfish
avocado	sweet potato	whiting
lemon	mushroom	clam
pineapple	green onion	haddock
tangerine	green bean	blue crab
sweet cherry	radish	trout
kiwi fruit	summer squash	halibut
lime	asparagus	lobster

More useful nutrition information is available from the Cancer Information Service at the National Cancer Institute. Call them at 1-800-422-6237.

The FDA Consumer, a magazine published by the Food and Drug Administration, often provides free reprints of timely articles on nutrition, diet and cancer treatment.

Research done on other countries and cultures frequently unearths excellent food sources unknown to Western society. A look at the diets and cancer rates in other cultures can be revealing.

WHAT CAN OTHER CULTURES TEACH US ABOUT DIET?

In 1990, Cornell University scientists completed one of the largest nutrition studies ever done: a comparison of Chinese and American eating habits. The seven-year study included 6,500 Chinese, who answered 367 questions about their daily eating habits. The study found:

1. Chinese eat 20 percent more calories than Americans, but are not as overweight

2. Chinese eat only one-third the amount of fat that Americans consume, and twice the number of starchy foods

3. Americans eat 33 percent more protein than Chinese; 70 percent of that from meat

4. Only seven percent of Chinese proteins come from meat

5. Chinese get most of their calcium from vegetable sources. Dairy products are rare in China, but so is osteoporosis

6. Chinese eat three times as much fiber as Americans

And while we are in China, it is interesting to note a National Cancer Institute study done at Linixian - an industrial city with a large incidence of stomach and esophagus cancers. Over five years, American researchers gave the following vitamins to a single group of Linixians. None of the vitamins has FDA approval as a cancer preventive, but they are known throughout the American lay and natural foods networks as cancer-fighters.

1. Retinol, a form of Vitamin A and zinc
2. Riboflavin and niacin, both B vitamins
3. Vitamin C and molybdenum, a form of yeast
4. Antioxidants: beta carotene, vitamin E and selenium

The study group that took the nutritional supplements suffered from fewer fatal cancers and degenerative diseases.

JAPAN'S ANTI-CANCER MUSHROOM

The National Cancer Institute is studying a Japanese fungus called a "Maitake," or "dancing mushroom." This rare, football-sized plant grows in rural northern Japan. Scientists purchased the mushroom in a powdered form to study its cancer-preventive reputation - it's called "dancing mushroom" because patients supposedly dance with joy after eating it.

The researchers found some truth to native claims - various forms and formulations stopped the growth of the HIV virus and certain cancer tumor cells. It also controls high blood pressure.

Because it is still under study, the FDA makes no claims about the maitake's health-giving effects. Those interested in more information on this fungus can contact Maitake Products of New Jersey at (201) 612-0097.

GREEN TEA

Green tea is one of the most popular drinks in Asia. Its naturally mild flavor comes from raw leaves that are not fermented - as opposed to most American teas. When you pour boiling water on green tea leaves, they double in size. What's more, Japanese scientists recently discovered a chemical component in green tea that lowers cholesterol and stops the growth of some cancers. It's called *epigallocatechin gallate* (EGCG), a substance that attacks cancer-producing "free radicals" in the body.

Free radicals - high-energy molecules - are present in every human body. However, too many may stimulate cancer growth. Free radicals are naturally controlled and destroyed by a balance of oxygen, fats, and elements in the body's immune system. Green tea "pumps up" the body's specialized immunity to free radicals, and thus may help prevent formation of cancerous tumors.

Dr. Fujiki, a researcher at the National Cancer Center Research Institute in Tokyo, said the average green tea drinker in Japan consumes a gram of EGCG per day. This may be one reason that Japanese have very low levels of lung cancer, even though they are among the world's heaviest smokers.

At Rutgers University's Laboratory for Cancer Research, Dr. Chung Yang gave green tea to mice infected with stomach and lung cancers. Incidence of the cancer dropped from 90 percent to 60 percent.

BETA-CAROTENE

Another powerful anti-cancer substance is found in the lowly carrot. Carrots are a super source of beta-carotene, an antioxidant that helps health problems like heart disease, cancer and cataracts. One study showed that the beta-carotene in one cup of carrots, taken daily, cuts the incidence of strokes in women by 40 percent and heart attacks by 22 percent.

Carrots are nature's richest source of beta-carotene. Beta-carotene is converted by the body to vitamin A. Studies show that those with high blood-levels of beta-carotene do not get cancer -and not only because of its link to vitamin A. Beta-carotene builds up the body's immune system. It is a powerful anti-oxidant, a substance that clears the body of cancer-causing free radicals.

The World Health Organization recommends the average 140 lb. adult consume up to 350 mg. of beta-carotene per day. Other government nutritionists recommend between 5 and 20 mgs. daily.

RISKY NUTRITION

FAT — It's easier than you might think to reduce your overall fat intake simply by making a few changes. Start by selecting lean cuts of meat. Remove the skin from chicken and other poultry before cooking and learn to love fish unbreaded, perhaps poached in a little court bullion (fish stock) for rich flavor. Use only low-fat dairy products and pass up pastries and other fat-loaded sweets. Another obvious benefit is that reducing fat in the diet helps keep weight down. A diet high in fat has been shown to increase the risk of breast, colon and prostate cancer.

Studies of various groups support this fact. For instance, the Japanese people traditionally eat a diet very low in fats in their homeland. But when they migrate to the U.S. and change their diet to correspond with western standards, their incidence of both breast and colon cancer rises dramatically. The death rate from cancer in America is five to ten times higher than in Japan.

Certain close-knit and health-conscious religious groups also exhibit a much lower incidence of cancer in general (and colon cancer in particular) than does the general population. The approximately 600,000 Seventh Day Adventists in the U.S. commonly eat a largely vegetarian diet which is also low in fats. A recent study showed that Seventh Day Adventists run a much lower risk of dying of colorectal cancers, smoke-related cancers, and breast cancer than a comparable group of nonmembers. The Mormons, although not strict vegetarians, follow a very healthy lifestyle. The use of tobacco, caffeinated beverages, and alcoholic spirits are forbidden. The Utah Cancer Registry has data which shows the incidence of lung, colorectal, breast, ovarian, and uterine cancer is far lower among Mormons than the national average. Interestingly, there is no difference in the incidence of prostate cancer in Mormon men than in the general population.

The scientists say that fat itself probably is not a primary cause of colon cancer, but instead nourishes the development of tumors caused by other substances. Fats increase the secretion of digestive juices (bile acids and steroids). It appears that the extra digestive chemicals needed to break down excessive fat intake may actually damage the walls of the intestines and thereby allow carcinogens to enter.

In breast cancer, a high fat diet contributes to obesity. The theory here is that carrying excess weight increases the body's production of the female hormone *estrogen,* which speeds up and fosters the growth of tumors.

An important fact to note in this context is that, as far as cancer development is concerned, it doesn't seem to matter what type of fat is consumed. Polyunsaturated fats are just as much a factor in cancer growth as are saturated fats, named by the American Heart Association as increasing the risk of heart disease because of their cholesterol content. Although the American Heart Association recommends polyunsaturates as preferable to saturated fats, both the American Cancer Society and the Heart Association are urging us to reduce our *total intake* of fats. The ACS says that only 30 percent of the day's calories should be consumed in fat. As things stand at this writing, the general public usually takes in more than 40 percent of the day's calories in fat. Both these prestigious agencies say that trimming away a mere 10 percent of fat from our daily meals will bring great benefits. (See Chapters 5 and 6.)

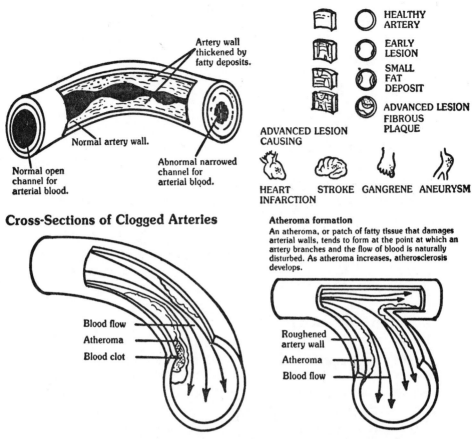

HEALTHY
ARTERY

EARLY
LESION

SMALL
FAT
DEPOSIT

ADVANCED LESION
FIBROUS
PLAQUE

ADVANCED LESION
CAUSING

HEART   STROKE   GANGRENE ANEURYSM
INFARCTION

Artery wall
thickened by
fatty deposits.

Normal artery wall.

Normal open
channel for
arterial blood.

Abnormal narrowed
channel for
arterial blood.

Cross-Sections of Clogged Arteries

Atheroma formation

An atheroma, or patch of fatty tissue that damages
arterial walls, tends to form at the point at which an
artery branches and the flow of blood is naturally
disturbed. As atheroma increases, atherosclerosis
develops.

Blood flow
Atheroma
Blood clot

Roughened
artery wall
Atheroma
Blood flow

CHOLESTEROL — Almost 30 percent of the nearly two
million deaths in the U.S. each year are caused by coronary
heart disease arising as a result of cholesterol-clogged arteries
that supply the heart. Over time, the arteries narrow, the flow
of blood is restricted, atherosclerosis develops, and a heart
attack occurs. Cholesterol is present in all foods of animal
origin and is part of every animal cell.

High serum cholesterol is one of the three major risk factors in coronary heart disease, but one you can control. (The
other two risk factors, which are fortunately also controllable,
are high blood pressure and cigarette smoking.) The experts
say that the typical American diet, high in saturated fats, raises
blood cholesterol levels. As serum cholesterol rises, the risk
of suffering a heart attack keeps pace and we are at additional
risk of developing certain forms of cancer as well.

Because the ingestion of cholesterol-producing saturated fats
has been officially labeled as being of great harm to the body,
this next statement may surprise you. *The body itself can*

59

manufacture cholesterol in quantities of about 1.5 grams daily. Cholesterol is the material the body uses to produce bile acids, certain hormones and provitamin D3. If cholesterol in the diet is reduced, the body goes into production and increases its manufacture. Studies indicate that diets deliberately kept low in cholesterol are often ineffective in reducing serum cholesterol levels in the blood because cholesterol is a fat. Like all fats, cholesterol is insoluble in water or blood. In order to transport it, the body transforms it into a lipoprotein (a combination of fat and protein). The trick is to keep the cholesterol in a liquid state so that it isn't deposited on arterial walls. The body does this very nicely when it's provided with the high-density lipoproteins (HDL) *lecithin* and *linoleic acid*. Interestingly enough, the very foods forbidden on a so-called low cholesterol diet (butter, milk, eggs, cheese, well-marbled beef), also contain more than enough HDL to keep cholesterol liquid and moving through the body.

The melting point of cholesterol itself is 300 degrees F. At the normal body temperature of 98.6 degrees, cholesterol ends up as a deposit on arterial walls, leading undeniably to atherosclerotic plaque. However, when lecithin, a saturated fatty acid, is supplied, the melting point of cholesterol comes down to 180 degrees, admittedly still insoluble at normal body temperature. But when a linoleate-containing dietary fat is supplied along with the lecithin, cholesterol liquifies at a cool 32 degrees F. These HDLs keep cholesterol liquid, the body absorbs what it needs, and no plaque accumulates on arterial walls to cause problems. Abracadabra! Why is it that some authorities think Mother Nature doesn't know what she's doing?

We are drifting a bit off center from our main subject of fats as they contribute to cancer, but you should know that a study of 900 men examined for signs of early atherosclerosis determined that those with more than 36 percent HDL in their blood had no atherosclerosis, but those with 34 percent or less HDL had evidence of the disease.

COMMERCIALLY PROCESSED FATS — Let's take a quick look at the process that brings us vegetable oils and margarine.

Vegetable seeds are crushed to release their oils and then put through a solvent (carbon tetrachloride or methylene chloride) to leach out the last bit of marketable oil. The resulting mess is then boiled to evaporate off as much of the chemical solvent as possible.

The next step is to remove whatever natural fatty acids remain, usually somewhere around 6 percent. The oil is cooked at temperatures of approximately 150 degrees F. with a solution of lye, producing an elementary type of soap which settles to the bottom of the witch's cauldron (processing chamber). The lighter oil is skimmed off, but the manufacturers still aren't satisfied.

Any so-called 'impurities' which remain (including important nutrients such as lecithin and carotene, a precursor of Vitamin A) are either filtered out through the same kind of adsorbent earth you use to clean your swimming pool or removed chemically. Placed in a vacuum, the oil is heated yet again to temperatures ranging as high as 380 degrees F. and held at temperature for at least 12 hours to completely deodorize it.

If the end product is to be a margarine, the manufacturer further subjects the oils to the hydrogenation process which alters the melting point to mimic the hardness of butter. Finally, an antioxidant (usually butylated hydroxyanisole) is added to extend shelf-life and the product ends up in the supermarket looking very attractive indeed.

Because the calorie count of the fat is not changed by all this chemical processing, the manufacturer can label the product accordingly. Unfortunately, nutritional scientists seem unaware that the resulting *unnatural* polyunsaturates possess as yet unknown biological properties. The one thing that *is* certain is that no natural nutrients remain. (See Chapter 5 for a detailed report on these destructive fats.)

Note: Only linseed (flax), pumpkin, soy, and walnut oils contain both essential fatty acids (linoleic and linolenic). The experts caution that these oils must be the cold-pressed, unrefined, natural varieties, and not the processed abominations found in most supermarkets. (See Chapters 5 and 6.)

NITROSAMINES — The American Cancer Society has determined that cancers of the esophagus and stomach are common in areas of the world where smoked, salt-cured, and nitrite-cured meats are eaten in large quantities. Many Americans find ham, bacon, sausage and hot dogs irresistible. These foods contain chemicals (nitrosamines and PAHs, polycyclic aromatic hydrocarbons) which cause cancer in animals. To be on the safe side, The American Cancer Society recommends that these foods, as well as salt-cured and smoked fish, be eaten only occasionally.

Nitrosamines are produced in the body from nitrites and nitrates used in curing certain foods. As an important additive in processing, these chemicals prevent the formation of deadly botulism spores which can cause death when they occur in foods. Unfortunately, the nitrosamines the body manufactures from foods cured in this manner are extremely carcinogenic.

Since this fact has become increasingly clear, science has been attempting to find ways to reduce the risk. It has been shown that Vitamin C can help prevent the body from manufacturing cancer-causing nitrosamines from nitrites. The meat industry is cooperating by adding Vitamin C to many chemically-cured products and has lowered their nitrite content as well. Does this render the foods completely safe? It will take more than a decade of studies before we know for sure.

A healthier method for handling these types of meat products, called 'The Wisconsin Process,' uses lactic acid in place of the harmful nitrites and nitrates. The discovery was announced in mid-1986, but don't look for meats processed by this method any time soon. The industry says it is cost-prohibitive.

Further, although the ACS does not include alcoholic beverages on their list of nitrosamine-containing foods, it is important to note here that some whiskies and all beers also contain nitrosamines. If alcoholic spirits are high on your list of priorities, you might want to consider switching to the colorless varieties, such as gin and vodka, which do not have nitrosamines. To round out the list of offending goodies in this category, we must also add pickled foods. Do you really need that fatty corned-beef sandwich with a dill pickle on the side?

FLAME BROILING — The luscious smoke-flavored meat barbecued over hot charcoal or wood coals (or gas) that's an entrenched part of Americana also poses a danger. When the fat melts and drips onto the coals, producing the smoke that so deliciously flavors the meat, it also produces potential carcinogens.

The PAH chemicals in the smoke that coat the meat are a very real threat to health. These compounds are similar to the tars inhaled by cigarette smokers. Authorities estimate that the quantity of harmful compounds we consume by eating just one flame-broiled steak is the same as if we sat down and smoked 600 cigarettes one after the other.

This information is not new. As long ago as 1775, a British scientist by the name of Sir Percival Pott discovered that chimney sweeps constantly exposed to the carbons in soot developed cancer. In the late 1800s, skin cancer in German laborers was tied to their work with coal tars. Coal tar is still used to produce cancer experimentally in laboratory animals.

SMOKED FOODS — Smoked foods, including lox (smoked salmon), other fishes, ham, poultry and cheeses, absorb PAHs during the curing process. The level of harmful compounds is lower in these processed foods than is created by direct flame broiling, but many smoked foods are also preserved by the addition of sodium nitrate (see above).

In areas of the world where smoked foods are commonly found on the menu, there are documented higher incidences of cancer. In both the U.S.S.R. and Iceland, where the populations are undeniably fond of smoked fish, gastric cancer rates in particular are extremely high.

MUTAGENS — Mutagens are not just something you find in a science fiction movie. A mutagen is any agent which is able to cause a change in the basic structure of genes. Many medicines, chemicals, and physical agents (radiation, ultraviolet light) have the ability to induce a genetic mutation. However, what we are primarily concerned with in this chapter are the carcinogenic mutagens which have been found in wide variety in cooked, smoked, roasted, and browned foods.

Research conducted by Dr. Barry Commoner at the Center for the Biology of Natural Substances, Washington University, revealed the presence of mutagens in coffee (roasted), hamburgers (as prepared in most fast-food facilities), and in many commercially processed foods. Commoner's research showed that meat developed mutagens when cooked at temperatures over 300 degrees F., as well as when the meat was in contact with metal for a long period.

Dr. Takashi Sugimura, a Japanese biologist, has determined that mutagens develop when the protein in food is heated. Dr. Sugimura has classified over a dozen mutagens produced when the proteins or amino acids are heated in the normal cooking process. Foods which produce mutagens in cooking include dairy products, cereals, potatoes, meat, fish and baked goods. Toasted bread (yes, our breakfast toast), french fried potatoes, black butter (named *beurre noire* in gourmet French cookery), and carmelized sugar all develop mutagens in the browning process. Science has yet to classify this type of mutagen as carcinogenic, but any substance able to do genetic damage is suspect. The experts say that the burned fat on roasted meat is another instance where the meat itself is bathed with potentially harmful chemicals as the fat melts and coats the meat during the roasting process. In addition, any overheated cooking oil which begins to smoke has developed harmful mutagens and should never be used to cook food.

PROTECT YOURSELF — If you insist on broiling meat, forego that flame-kissed flavor. The experts say that when the heat source comes from above the meat and not below it, the risk of ingesting the harmful chemical compounds is minimized. When the heat radiates down on the meat, the browning fat drips into the broiler pan. The fat thus does not sizzle and flame and the smoke which carries the carcinogenic hydrocarbons (PAHs) does not occur.

Washington University has determined that broiling meat under an electric element or using a microwave (without a browning plate) will reduce health risks dramatically. Meats cooked in this manner did not develop mutagens.

More good news is the fact that experimental studies show that when green vegetables are eaten at the same meal as fried/flame-broiled meat, a significantly reduced number of mutagens are excreted in the urine, indicating that the mutagens in the meat are neutralized to some degree by ingesting vegetables at the same time. After a meal of fried meat alone, mutagenic levels in the body are increased. This fact has been confirmed by urinalysis. This study clearly indicates that certain foods can protect against potentially carcinogenic heat-induced mutagens.

Therefore, science makes a strong case for serving and eating greens with any basic meat dish. Essential fatty acids (linoleic and linolenic), present in abundance in *unrefined* virgin linseed, pumpkin, soy, and walnut oils, plus certain antioxidants (Vitamins C and E, selenium), not only protect against mutagens, but against cancer as well. Along with the important vitamins, strong antimutagenic substances have been identified in wheat sprouts, leaf lettuce, brussel sprouts, mustard greens, cabbage, broccoli, and spinach. Popeye knew it all the time.

ALTERNATIVE NUTRITIONAL APPROACHES TO CANCER PROTECTION

The 1990 *Cancer Facts and Figures,* a publication of the American Cancer Society, lists diet as a "primary cancer protection." Nutritional approaches to cancer prevention - and treatment - aim to build up the body through good nutrition and rid the system of accumulated toxins. The following therapies use this approach to restore the body's natural immunity to cancer.

WHEATGRASS THERAPY

Wheat grass is grown from wheatberries or wheat seeds, substances rich in chlorophyll, which resembles the hemoglobin in human blood. Chlorophyll is the green protein pigment found in plants. It acts as a carrier, transporting oxygen to plant cells. Wheat grass, rich in chlorophyll, is also packed with oxygen.

Wheat plants used for medicinal purposes are cut while still very young. They are pressed naturally, and yield a sweet, green juice that contains more than 100 vitamins and minerals, all eight amino acids and many other essential nutrients. Wheatgrass has more vitamin C than oranges and more iron than spinach. Enzymes essential for cell functions and blood cleansing are also found in this anti-cancer wheat. Noted cancer-fighting substances absidic acid and laetrile - vitamin B17 - are also abundant in wheatgrass.

Wheatgrass therapy was brought to the United States by Ann Wigmore, a Lithuanian woman, in the 1960s. The grass had been used for decades in Europe as a dietary supplement. For centuries previous the grass was grown in India, where naturopathic health clinics treated cancer patients with a diet of raw vegetables, fruits and plants grown in soil free from pesticides and chemical fertilizers.

THE WHEATGRASS REGIME

Wigmore's wheatgrass therapy for cancer patients begins with a thorough detoxification of the body systems, beginning with a three-day juice fast. The diet includes wheatgrass juice, which many patients grow and squeeze at their homes. (It is also available at many health food stores.) They also consume plenty of fruit juice, lemon water and "Rejuvelac," a fermented drink made from wheatberries and the "friendly" milk bacteria found in natural yogurt.

Throughout the fast, patients undergo "colonics" - a series of therapeutic enemas. Both water and wheatgrass are taken deep into the bowel once or twice a day. Wheatgrass nutrients can also be absorbed directly through the walls of the colon.

Wigmore explains the procedure in "The Wheatgrass Book:"

> "(Wheatgrass enemas) are excellent for loosening hard fecal matter. The high magnesium content of

wheatgrass is particularly effective for drawing out toxins from not only the colon but the liver and kidneys. Wheatgrass is also beneficial for supplying the body with missing nutrients, because the soluble ingredients from the wheatgrass juice can be absorbed by the portal circulation inside the colon. Most important, though, is the fact that you are introducing one of the most concentrated energies of the life force and sun into one of the most diseased areas of your body."

Ann Wigmore learned about wheatgrass's health benefits when she was a child. She was raised by her grandmother, the town "healer," in a small Eastern European village. Ann grew up on a diet of herbs, roots, grasses, goat milk and bread made of rye and straw.

During the turmoil of World War I, Ann, her grandmother and a few others lived through a winter in an orchard cellar, eating roots and grasses. At age 16, Ann emigrated to the United States. She studied naturopathic medicine, but adopted the native diet of fried foods, refined sugar, meat and fat. She got sick - she says her body responded to its new diet by developing colon cancer and gangrene.

A hasty return to the rough-and-raw diet of her grandmother healed her disease, Ann says. After years of study and writing for a national nutrition magazine, Ann began to study the benefits of wheatgrass. She consulted with Dr. Earp Thomas, a soil scientist, whose analysis of the grass found more than 100 nutritional elements.

Ann first experimented with the effects of wheatgrass on newly hatched chicks. A portion of chicks that received wheatgrass as well as a regular feed developed more feathers and was heavier and more alert than chicks fed a regular diet, she found. Similar effects were noticed in experiments on rabbits and cats.

It was a small step to human use of the wheatgrass. In 1963, Wigmore founded the Hippocrates Health Institute in Boston, an organization that promotes self-healing techniques. Many wheatgrass health clinics have sprung up since then throughout the United States, most with the name "Hippocrates" attached.

In the 1930s, Nobel Prize winner Otto Warburg, a biochemist, discovered that cancer cells cannot grow in the presence of oxygen. Warburg found that cell mutation occurs in an environment of oxygen deprivation. Warburg's ideas are proven true when we look at the rise in modern cancer cases and the inactivity of modern lifestyles. Air pollution, smoking, fat and protein consumption and sedentary lifestyles all reduce the body's oxygen levels.

Way back then, Warburg said any cancer therapy must increase the amount of oxygen carried to body cells. Wheatgrass therapy does just that. Rich in chlorophyll, wheatgrass juice helps improve blood circulation, which nourishes the cells.

Japanese scientist and doctor Yoshihide Hagiwara frequently prescribes grasses as medicine for his patients. He claims that chlorophyll can be directly absorbed into the bloodstream through the lymphatic system.

Other Japanese scientists associated with Hagiwara discovered the amino acids and enzymes found in wheatgrass, deactivated the cancer-causing effects of benzyprene - the dangerous substance found in charcoal-broiled meats and smoked fish.

Dr. Tsuneo Kada, director of the Japanese Research Center of Genetics, found the juice of green plants stops chromosome damage - a major step a cell undergoes in the process of becoming cancerous. The enzymes in the green grass efficiently rid the body of toxins and the ill effects of pollution.

More wheatgrass research was done by Dr. Chiu-Nan Lai, a University of Texas biologist. Lai showed that extracts from roots and leaves of wheat sprouts have an antimutagenic effect - they decrease abnormal cell mutation. This is what occurs in cancer: abnormal cells mutate,

68

then multiply. Lai also showed that the wheat-sprout extracts destroyed cancer tumors without the toxic effects of most chemotherapy drugs.

TESTIMONIES OF WHEATGRASS PATIENTS

Prospects weren't good for David Jones of Vancouver, British Columbia. He had incurable cancer. A three-inch tumor had wrapped around his backbone and entered his spinal column. This erstwhile athlete started wheatgrass therapy in January, 1989, but was completely paralyzed when he entered the hospital four weeks later.

Doctors removed the tumor. Jones refused follow-up radiation and chemotherapy treatments. Four days after his surgery, he walked out of the hospital, using only a cane. The doctors were amazed.

By early 1990, David was swimming and riding his mountain bike again. He made two trips to Boston to learn the details of Ann Wigmore's therapy. In August his doctor found no trace of cancer in his body - the cancer was in remission.

David says he is grateful for the surgery that removed the tumor, but he's glad he followed the wheatgrass therapy. He plans to write a book on his experience.

"You don't get well by pouring juice down your throat," David says. "Wheatgrass therapy is a complete lifestyle, involving what and how you eat, and the way you think and feel about yourself."

Marianne Dimetres of Southwick, Massachusetts combined wheatgrass therapy, vitamins and surgery to send her uterine cancer into remission. In 1988, Marianne was diagnosed with Stage 4 cancer of the uterus. Her doctor advised immediate surgery, but instead she spent three weeks at the Hippocrates Health Institute in Florida, undergoing an intensive wheatgrass regimen.

"By the end of the visit, I felt better than I'd felt in years," Marianne said. "The Wheatgrass therapy was part of a program that turned my life around. It reduced the pain and pressure, and helped improve my bloodwork. I had lost my voice due to growths on my vocal cords, but the wheatgrass therapy helped me regain my voice within a few months." After she returned home, she continued the wheatgrass therapy.

Marianne later underwent surgery. Her uterus and part of her abdominal wall were removed, but doctors found the tumors on her ovaries and fallopian tubes were gone. By 1991, the cancer was in remission.

"I really do believe that conventional medicine has its place in treatment," Marianne affirmed. "But I also believe that you should have control of your own healing and freedom to choose what's best for you. Getting well is not just a question of taking medicine. It's a life choice. It involves your body, mind and spirit."

Those interested in referrals or further information can contact:

The Ann Wigmore Foundation
196 Commonwealth Ave.
Boston, MA 02116
(619) 267-9424

For details on wheatgrass therapy contact:

Hippocrates Health Institute
1443 Palmdale Court
West Palm Beach, FL 33411
(407) 471-8876

RUDOLPH STEINER'S ANTI-CANCER THERAPY

Rudolph Steiner, a European biological researcher discovered more than romance under the mistletoe. He found that an extract made from the familiar plant increases immune system activity and stops cancer cells from

70

growing. It does this by stimulating the thymus gland, which regulates immunity.

Steiner called his anti-cancer extract "Iscador." This fermented extract was studied closely in 1990. Scientists found that cultures of human cells produced more anti-tumor hormones when they were treated with a mistletoe protein. Since then, some clinics have adopted Iscador for treatment of cancer.

A few warnings are in order for the herbal enthusiast eager to experiment. Steiner's extract is made from European mistletoe plants. Mistletoe berries are poisonous, so never eat them. The stems and leaves must be processed before using as medicine; and the finished product raises blood pressure and pulse: those with heart problems should not use it. Also, patients taking anti-depressant medications containing monoamine oxidase should avoid Iscador. Mixing these two compounds causes serious side effects.

Steiner and his associates offer a full therapy of Iscador and other treatments at the Lukas Klinik, a Swiss spa. Treatments include a special vegetarian diet, herbs, and forms of art and movement therapy.

You may contact the Lukas Klinik by writing:

Lukas Klinik
4144 Arlesheim
Switzerland
Phone 011-41-61-701-3333

For information on U.S. physicians who utilize mistletoe extract, contact:

Physicians Association for Anthroposophical Medicine
PO Box 269
Kimberton, PA 19442

ALTERNATIVE CANCER TREATMENTS

IMMUNE THERAPIES

The immune system is the body's first line of defense against all kinds of disease and illness. In even a slight sprain, the body responds in a way that will prevent further injury. It pools all the body's resources to heal the wounded area.

But with cancer and immune deficiency diseases like AIDS, the body's defense system stops behaving in a healing manner. With cancer, the body appears to feed the cancer tumor at the expense of the rest of the body. The precious nutrients the body so desperately needs are drained away. The patient becomes malnourished, while the cancer thrives.

Immune therapies aim at strengthening the part of the immune system that fights and destroys cancer cells. Cancerous cells are created inside every body, but a strong, healthy immune system usually destroys them before they can multiply.

But sometimes, the immune system fails to recognize the cancer as a foreign invader. The cancer slowly grows, without the patient showing warning signs of disease. After five or ten years symptoms appear - after the cancer has reached a stage of rapid growth.

What causes the immune system to ignore cancer cells? Researchers hold several theories as to how and why cancer develops. Reasons include poor nutrition, stress, smoking, air and water pollution, toxic chemicals in our food, water and clothing. Some factors are more easily controlled than others.

Normally, the immune system is on constant alert. It patrols the body for bacteria, viruses, or abnormal cells. It employs antigens - special "killer cells," specialized to kill off foreign substances.

If cancer overwhelms this first level of defense, the injured antigens the cancer cells leave behind are detected by t-cells. T-cells, also called t-lymphocytes, destroy cancerous cells and cells infected with viruses. These special white blood cells are produced in the bone marrow and processed through the thymus gland in the brain.

Macrophages are another type of white blood cell that actually consumes cancer cells. Numerous other types of white blood cells work together to destroy cancerous renegades.

Doctors use five major types of orthodox immunotherapy, but they are very toxic and produce a wide array of negative side effects. They are:

BCG: This tuberculin vaccine programs the macrophages to kill off cancer cells. This appears to work well with chemotherapy, and is especially useful in treating skin cancer.

INTERFERON: This is a group of related proteins manufactured by white blood cells in response to a virus. Interferon triggers production of macrophages, which attack cancer cells and block tumor growth. It transforms some lymph cells into "cancer killers." When Interferon was first introduced, it was hailed as a medical miracle. Its side effects and high cost have tarnished its appeal, however.

INTERLEUKIN-2: This is another protein manufactured by t-cells. It attacks cancer cells, but its side effects often outweigh its benefits. Users report chills, bleeding, swelling of the spleen, shock and confusion.

TUMOR NECROSIS FACTOR (TNF): This is a cancer cell killer produced by the body; doctors still do not understand how it is produced or how it works. Side effect include flu-like symptoms.

MONOCLONAL ANTIBODIES: These are sythetically produced antibodies manufactured through gene splicing. A cancer patient's own white blood cells are combined in a laboratory dish with cancer cells, and are then returned to the body. The combination works as an antigen, attacking only cancer cells. These would, hypothetically, work like guided missiles, with the cancer as a target. As wonderful as this therapy sounds, it is still in the experimental stage. When and if it becomes a treatment standard it will no doubt be very costly.

STAPHE LYSATE: is a vaccine made from staphylococci. It is used for allergies, asthma, herpes, multiple sclerosis and cancer. It is non-toxic and inexpensive, and can be taken orally, injected or inhaled to encourage the body to produce interferon, t-cells and interleukin-1.

The American Cancer Society says it will take many years for scientists to find the proper role of these orthodox immunotherapies in cancer treatments. However, there are alternative immunotherapies under study that have helped many cancer patients. These include Livingston Therapy and the Issel Whole Body Approach.

THE LIVINGSTON THEORY

The Livingston Anti-Cancer Therapy, pioneered by Dr. Virginia Livingston, MD, is based on a bacterial theory of cancer. Dr. Livingston claims cancer is caused by a form-changing microbe she discovered in 1947 and named "progenitor cryptocite:" or "ancestral killer." Dr. Livingston repeatedly isolated this microbe from every laboratory cancer sample she analyzed, both human and animal. She observed that animals injected with this form-changing bacteria developed cancer soon after. She also isolated the bacteria in human sperm cells.

Dr. Livingston believes this "progenitor" is in everyone from birth to death, and is held in check by the immune system. When the immune system is weakened by stress, poor nutrition, surgery, toxins or other cancer-causing substances, these microbes multiply and promote tumor growth. Doctors find large numbers of these "progenitor" microbes in all cancer patients. Using an electron microscope, Dr. Livingston and her associates discovered the bacteria can change into a virus-like form.

74

Many scientists don't believe these form-changing germs exist. When they are shown them under a microscope, many doctors dismiss them as "unexplainable anomalies." Livingston says these germs adapt to their environment by shedding their cell walls and dispersing among body tissues, waiting for opportunity to revert to their original forms.

Dr. Raymond Brown, MD, a former fellow at the Memorial Sloan-Kettering Institute for Cancer Research, said these organisms are "demonstrable as the silent stage of a gamut of infections. They have repeatedly been found in cancer, arthritis, multiple sclerosis and other diseases of undetermined origin."

LIVINGSTON THERAPY

The goal of Livingston therapy is restoration of the body's natural defenses by strengthening the immune system. Her regime includes vaccines, a vegetable and raw foods diet, gamma globulin, vitamin and mineral supplements, antibodies and autogenous vaccines made from a culture of the patient's own bacteria.

HOW CAN A BACTERIA CAUSE A MALIGNANT TUMOR?

Dr. Livingston and her associates posit that P. cryptocides attack the genetic "memory" inside cells, causing healthy cells to suddenly multiply uncontrollably. William Diller, MD, microbiologist with the Institute for Cancer Research in Philadelphia, has found cancer microbes interfering with normal cell division, producing strange, precancerous cell abnormalities.

And in 1974, Livingston's researchers found these microbes secrete a hormone almost identical to human chorionic gonadotropin (HCG) - the substance that protects fetus and placenta from a mother's immune system. In the same way, this hormone protects the cancer cell from detection by the body's immune system.

75

Sadly, Livingston's discovery of the growth hormone wasn't taken seriously until scientists at Rockefeller University, Princeton Laboratory and Allegheny General Hospital in Pittsburgh isolated it in lab samples.

Dr. Livingston found that abscisic acid, a substance found in plant hormones and vitamin A, neutralizes the production of HCG. She called abscisic acid "nature's most potent anti-cancer weapon," and noted that all cancer patients have very low abscisic acid levels. This acid stops cancer cell multiplication, and shrinks tumors in laboratory animal tests.

Naturally, Livingston's diet contributes large doses of vitamin A. She warns, however, that simply consuming large amounts of vitamins isn't enough to prevent or stop cancer.

"Certain malnourished people, and nearly all cancer patients, have lost the ability to break down vitamin A in their livers," Livingston said. "So I have included a table of foods which are high in abscisins."

THE LIVINGSTON DIET

Dr. Livingston has her cancer patients eat plenty of raw fruits and vegetables. She also prescribes the following foods, which are high in abscisic acid:

cauliflower	mangoes	avocadoes
tomatoes	lima beans	leafy green vegetables
potatoes	dwarf peas	yams
sweet potatoes	asparagus	onions
spinach	grapes	tangerines
pears	nuts	strawberries
oranges	kale	chard
lentils	soy beans	mustard greens
celery	endive	bananas
comfrey	cabbage	beet greens
corn	large lettuce	romaine lettuce
apricots	papaya	melons
grapefruit	apples	

76

Use these fruit blossoms and their leaves in tea:

peach flowers   apple blossoms   strawberry leaves
cherry flowers

Eat plenty of root vegetables like carrots, turnips, radishes, kohlrabi, artichokes, beets and rutabagas.

Whole grains and breads are also important. These include:

wheat flakes	brown rice	millet
rye flakes	buckwheat	oats
bulgur	rye	open-pollinated corn
barley	triticale	whole wheat

Livingston usually has patients eat raw foods whenever possible, because vitamin A is destroyed if the food is heated over 275 degrees F - the average temperature for steaming and boiling.

The doctor also has patients drink carrot juice and take supplements of dried liver powder. Liver enzymes break down the vitamin A in the carrot juice, and contribute to production of retinoids - the anti-cancer substances the patient needs to build up his immune system. As the doctor says: "If you do not have the retinoic acids, you cannot build up immunity. It's that simple."

At her clinic, Dr. Livingston offers three diets: a strict regimen for the seriously ill; a recuperation diet; and a maintenance diet for those who've recovered. Sample meals are as follows:

STRICT CANCER DIET

BREAKFAST:

> 8 oz. carrot juice with a quarter pureed avocado stirred in
> millet with nut cream
> whole grain toast
> violet leaf tea
> prescribed supplements

LUNCH:

> garden salad with grated carrot and horseradish dressing
> black bean soup
> curried vegetables
> choice of raw squash, okra, zucchini, celery carrots,
> turnip or parsnip slices
> whole grain bread and sweet butter
> strawberry leaf tea
> prescribed supplements

DINNER:

> garden salad
> cream of mushroom soup
> spaghetti squash
> whole grain bread and sweet butter
> peppermint leaf tea

More such menus, shopping lists, recipes and recommendations are listed in Livingston's book "The Conquest of Cancer," available at any good book store.

RUDOLPH BREUSS'S CANCER THEORY AND TREATMENT

Rudolph Breuss was an Austrian herbalist and naturopath who successfully treated many cancer patients using a special healing fast. Breuss made his knowledge public in 1982, when, at age 82, he published his book "Advice for the Prevention and Natural Treatment of Numerous Diseases."

Breuss' natural treatment is very intense. He insisted that patients strictly follow his treatment to ensure its effectiveness. Patients who have received high doses of radiation or chemotherapy may not respond to the treatment, but all others were encouraged to give it a try.

Breuss believed that fasting triggers the body to purge itself of all foreign materials - including cancers. He viewed cancer as an autonomous growth, something that is not really a part of the patient's system. Using juice and herbal teas will sometimes encourage the body to simply consume and eliminate tumors, he said.

Dr. F.B. Berchtesgaden, a Breuss contemporary, witnessed the healing of many cancer patients through Breuss' methods. He wrote: "There is no other way we will overcome cancer other than the pharmaceutical branch of the chemical industry finding a remedy similar to the one used for tuberculosis. The body, though, would have to be strong to stand the chemical treatment. There is always an element of risk involved in new drugs. It is, therefore, always better to try natural herbs to fight cancer."

BREUSS THEORY OF CANCER DEVELOPMENT

Breuss believed that cancer develops from exposure to many environmental factors - daily consumption of over-cooked foods, repeated contact with cloth dyes, smoke or hazardous materials on the job or at home. Patients often don't suspect they have a problem until the cancer has reached an advanced stage. By the time a lump or other symptom appears, metabolic deterioration may have been ongoing for up to ten years.

Breuss believed that unnatural pressure on body parts cuts blood flow to specific spots, which causes cancerous cells to form. In an attempt to survive, the cells in the affected area try to draw supplies from surrounding, healthy cells. The newly formed tumor then uses this supply line to feed itself at the expense of surrounding tissue. It grows slowly at first, and after a number of years "takes off."

BREUSS' NINE CANCER WARNING SIGNS

1. Tangible lumps, especially in the breast or groin
2. Changes on birthmarks or nipples
3. Changes in bowel or bladder habits
4. Persistent sore throats or coughing

5. Difficulty swallowing, especially among the elderly

6. Heavy, abnormal bleeding from any body orifice

7. Wounds that will not heal

8. Swellings that will not go down

9. Noticeable weight gain or loss

(These warning signs are also outlined in the National Cancer Institute's "Cancer Facts" booklet.)

At the onset of any of these symptoms, Breuss would have his patients begin his "total cancer treatment."

Breuss taught that cancer growths feed on protein - proteins found in solid foods. He claimed that his diet, strictly followed for 42 days, will kill the cancer tumor and spare the patient's life. Without protein, cell growth cannot occur. Healthy cells begin to feel the pinch of starvation, and then attack fluid parts of the body like growths, waste matter and swollen areas. Breuss saw this as a natural process, in which "the blood accomplishes its purpose."

TOTAL CANCER TREATMENT

Taking the Breuss cure isn't easy. For 42 days you cannot eat anything but vegetable juice (see below), and the corresponding teas on the following pages, in specific amounts. Patients can drink the Basic Breuss Juice when hungry, but not more than 1/2 quart over a period of one day. The less you drink, the better.

HOW TO PREPARE THE BREUSS VEGETABLE JUICES FOR TREATMENT:

8 oz. red beet root   1 oz. radish
3 oz. carrots   1 small potato (peeled)
3 oz. celery root

The potato is only absolutely necessary in cases of liver cancer.

Press the vegetables into a food processor and liquefy, or use a juicer instead. Put the juice through a sieve or linen towel to strain. (If a juicer is used, you don't have to put juice through a sieve or linen towel.)

Those who dislike the flavor or texture of the potato can omit it from the juice mixture and, instead, drink a cup of potato peel tea per day. (To make this appealing drink, cook a handful of potato peelings in 2 cups of boiling water for 2 to 4 minutes.)

Beets provide the key cancer-fighting ingredient in the diet, Breuss said. Carrots and celery are added to provide needed nutrients.

HOW TO PREPARE HERBAL TEAS FOR TREATMENT

Three herbal tea mixtures provide another important aspect in the Breuss therapy.

1) *Kidney Tea:*

Horsetail (equisetum arvense)	1 tsp.
Nettle (urtica dioica)	1/2 tsp.
Knot grass (polygonum aviculare) packed down	1/4 tsp.
St. Johnswort (hypericum perforatum)	1/8 tsp.

No sugar or sweeteners of any kind allowed.

Take a pinch of the tea mixture between thumb and two fingers and steep in 1 cup of hot water for 10 minutes. Strain liquid off and set it aside. Then pour two cups of hot water over the wet tea mixture again and boil for 10 minutes. Strain out the tea mixture and combine the first cup of tea with the two remaining. The reason for this is because of an important ingredient, *silicic acid* , which can only be extracted through boiling.

This mixture will last for 3 weeks for one person. Store in airtight container.

Kidney Tea is strong medicine, and should only be taken for 3 weeks. Drink 1/2 cup of tea before breakfast (on an empty stomach), before lunch and before bedtime.

After using for three weeks, discontinue for 2 or 3 weeks, and then resume taking the tea again. During this time, refrain from eating soup with meat and do not eat any beef or pork.

2) *Sage Tea (salvia officinalis):*

Take 1 to 2 teaspoons of sage and put in 1/2 quart of boiling water and boil for 3 minutes. Then set aside, and add immediately a small pinch of St. Johnswort (hyperocum perforatum), balm (melissa officinalis) and peppermint (mentha piperita). The oil in the leaves will boil away, but the enzymes are released. These are important elements to the glands and spinal cord.

2a) *Sage Tea (salvia officinalis):*

For gargling:

Sage contains an essential oil which is important when you gargle, but you are *not* allowed to swallow or drink this. Simply soak 2 teaspoons in 2 cups of hot water for 10 minutes.

3) *Cranesbill Tea (geranium robertianum):*

Add a pinch of cranesbill tea to one cup of hot water and soak for 10 minutes. Drink one cup of cold tea per day, little by little.

THE TOTAL BREUSS TREATMENT -
CONSISTING OF THE VEGETABLE JUICES AND HERBAL TEAS

Early morning:

Slowly drink 1/2 cup cold kidney tea.

30 to 60 minutes later:

Drink 1 or 2 cups warm sage tea mixed with small amounts of St. Johnswort, peppermint and balm. (See recipe above for preparation of tea.)

30 to 60 minutes later:

Take a small mouthful of juice mixture, but do not swallow it right away. Salivate, then swallow slowly.

15 to 30 minutes later:

Take a small amount of vegetable juice, or more according to your hunger. Always hold it in your mouth and allow yourself to salivate before slowly swallowing.

Mid mornings:

> You may take 10 or 15 very small sips of juice if you so desire. Accompany this with cold sage tea, *unsugared* , as much as you like.

After lunchtime:

> Drink 1/2 cup of kidney tea.

Before bedtime:

> Drink 1/2 cup of kidney tea.

Kidney tea should be taken for only 3 weeks out of the 42 days. After 3 weeks, you may take, instead of Kidney tea, small sips of the vegetable juice if you so desire, but not more than 1/2 quart per day. *It is very important that you always use the vegetable juices according to the recipe, in connection with the appropriate teas. Swallow in small amounts only and salivate well. Never drink only vegetable juice, but also the teas as recommended.*

SPECIAL TEAS FOR SPECIFIC CANCERS -
WHICH SHOULD BE TAKEN ALONG WITH THE TOTAL BREUSS TREATMENT

CEREBRAL TUMOR:

> To brew, steep a pinch of balm (melissa officinalis) in a cup of hot water for 10 minutes. Slowly drink one or two cups of cold balm tea per day, little by little.

BREAST CANCER:

> Brew a pinch of silvery lady's mantle tea (alchemilla alpina) and lady's mantle tea (alchemilla vulgaris) mixed with a pinch of blind nettle (laminum album) in a cup of hot water for 10 minutes, and drink cold little by little during the day.

SKIN CANCER:

> The juice of celandine (chelidonum majus) is useful as an anti-cancer swab. Peel the herb until you see a yellow, buttery juice appear; spread this on the affected skin once a day. If the spot is large, apply only to the part touching healthy skin.

CANCER OF THE GUMS, MOUTH, TONGUE, NECK OR LARYNX:

Use a gargle of pimpernel tea (pimpinella saxifraga) and use for 42 days. To brew, place a teaspoon of pimpernel root tea in water and boil for three minutes. To use, gargle a tablespoonful two times, and spitting out each. Take a third spoonful, gargle, then swallow. This can be repeated a few times during the day.

CANCER OF THE BONES AND LUNGS:

Blend together equal small amounts of common plantain (plantago lanceolata, plantago major) Iceland moss (cetraria islandica) lungwort (pulmonaria officinalis) ground ivy (nepeta hederacea) and orange mullein (verbascum phlomoides). Steep for 10 minutes in hot water and drink as much as you like, the more the better.

CANCER OF THE SPLEEN OR PANCREAS:

Drink at least a quart of sage tea daily, warm or cold.

PROSTATE AND TESTICLE CANCER:

Drink two cups of cold small-flowered willow herb tea each day in small quantities. To brew, put a pinch of the herb in a cup of hot water and steep for 10 minutes.

LIVER CANCER:

Take a handful of raw potato peels and brew in 2 cups of hot water for 2 to 4 minutes. Drink two cups a day, warm or cold. Breuss said "If this tea tastes good to you, then your liver needs it! If it tastes bad, you should not drink it."

CONSTIPATION:

If constipation should occur, this can be remedied by taking enemas with warm chamomile tea or you can drink a mild aperient tea.

According to Rudolph Breuss, cancer cells cannot develop and thrive on vegetable juices and teas (if taken for 42 days) they can only thrive on solid food. He has proven this theory on over 40,000 patients who have all been cured from this deadly disease.

Breuss' patients stand willing to testify to the healthy effects of this rigorous diet. Mrs. M.N. from Bludenz, Austria, recovered from breast cancer after 42 days of Breuss' therapy in 1950. In 1982, she was still cancer-free.

Olga Marte, German, was diagnosed with cancer of the stomach and bowel. She decided to try the Breuss treatment in lieu of surgery. She said it wasn't an easy diet - she didn't have a juice press! But after losing 22 pounds and fasting 40 days, the cancer "discharged itself through my bowels," she said. Twenty-five years later, she's had no relapses.

Breuss advised patients who've finished their full 42-day fasts to only slowly start eating solid foods again. The juice mixture should continue as part of the diet for two to four weeks after - 1/2 cup per day is recommended - swallowed slowly before meals. He advised supplementing the recovery period with vitamin elixirs and Brewer's Yeast tablets.

Breuss said he treated about 2,000 patients with the fast - not all of them afflicted with cancer. Many of his most successful cases were elderly, frail folk, who nevertheless seemed to thrive on this Spartan diet.

BREUSS' JUICE AND THE FDA

Breuss' therapies are 30 years old, but the Federal Food & Drug Administration is now discovering the wisdom of his prescriptive. Way back then, Breuss taught that diet and nutrition effect cancer.

In 1992, the National Cancer Institute announced with fanfare that Americans concerned about cancer should eat five servings of fresh fruits and vegetables each day.

In 1993, the Department of Agriculture listed in "The FDA Consumer" the top 20 fruits and vegetables, based on nutritional value and cancer-fighting properties.

They were the same food items Breuss' patients were told to eat. Over the past ten years, researchers have uncovered the healing properties of Beta-carotene, plant fiber and vitamin C - all of them abundant in the fruit juices, teas and fresh, whole foods this herbalist prescribed for years.

OTHER IMPORTANT "CANCER-CONSCIOUS" FOODS
THE CABBAGE FAMILY

The cabbage family includes broccoli, cauliflower, mustard greens and brussels sprouts as well as cabbage. All contain indole, a substance that destroys inactive estrogen in the human bloodstream. Inactive estrogen is known to initiate new cancers - especially breast cancer.

Researchers at Rockefeller University discovered the positive effects of indole on estrogen. The scientists fed the substance to healthy human volunteers. Blood tests showed that after seven days, their estrogen levels had decreased by up to 50 percent.

Cabbage helps the body get rid of toxic drugs and carcinogens. Laboratory tests found cabbage juice stops bacterial mutations and protect against low-level radiation, too.

A Cornell University study showed that laboratory rats fed brussels sprouts did not develop induced breast cancer tumors. Cancers in rats previously infected went into remission after six weeks of a brussels sprout diet.

Nutritionists believe cabbage contains numerous antioxidant and anti-cancer compounds. Studies found that foods from the cabbage family suppress colon polyps - the precursors of colon cancer. Men who eat cabbage more than once a week can cut their colon cancer odds by 66 percent!

ORANGES AND CITRUS

Oranges and citrus fruits are a complete package of cancer inhibitors. Oranges are tied to lower pancreatic cancer rates. Their high vitamin C content may ward off breast and stomach cancers as well.

The healing power of vitamin C has been known since the 1700s, when British sailors found they didn't suffer from scurvy - a bone disease - if they took limes and lemons along on lengthy voyages. (And thus the nickname "limey" for the English seaman!)

In 1920, Hungarian scientist Albert Szent-Gyorgyi isolated vitamin C from paprika and won the Nobel Prize for his discovery. Modern scientists continue to tout the positive effects of citrus. Two-time Nobel winner Dr. Linus Pauling argues that large doses of vitamin C can effect the occurrence of colds and their severity.

And research conducted at the National Cancer Institute found that vitamin C is effective in treating cancer. They found that mice with skin cancer lived just as long on a vitamin C supplement as mice given a cancer drug.

In 1990, the National Cancer Institute sponsored a symposium on Ascorbic Acid (vitamin C) and its functions in relation to cancer. About 130 doctors heard presentations by 40 research teams. Significant findings included:

From the University of California, Berkeley: Dr. Balz Frei said he considers vitamin C "the most effective anti-oxidant in human blood plasma." Frei's research showed that some of the chemical reactions that cause cancer cannot occur with vitamin C present.

From the University of Tokyo, Dr. E. Niki said that cancer-causing free radicals are destroyed faster by vitamin C than by any other antioxidant.

Dr. Linus Pauling and Dr. Abram Hoffer, a well-known Canadian biochemist and psychiatrist, worked together on a study of vitamin C and cancer in women. A "control group" of 11 women with cancers of the breast, ovaries or fallopian tubes were treated with standard therapies. All but one died within five months - the remaining woman was very ill. Of the group given supplemental vitamin C, half were alive and all but two were rated "very well."

The doctors concluded that cancer patients should take vitamin C in addition to conventional cancer therapies.

From the University of Texas, Dr. Joachim Liehr reported that vitamin C inhibits growth of estrogen-related kidney tumors. He treated hamsters with vitamins C, which later proved to protect them against shots of a synthetic cancer-causing hormone.

Dr. Gladys Block of the National Cancer Institute summarized the conference thus: Of the 46 studies read, 33 showed that vitamin C consumed in foods protects living tissue from cancer. Those with high vitamin C levels were half as likely to develop cancer.

Of 29 studies that focused on fruit, 21 showed it lends a significant portion of cancer protection. Cancers of the esophagus, larynx, mouth and pancreas showed especially marked responses to vitamin C. She concluded that science upholds the old wisdom: eating a combination of fresh fruits and vegetables has a positive effect on cancer prevention.

GARLIC:

While hunter-gatherers cultivated their first garlic bulbs in the Middle East about 5,000 years ago, western Russians were pounding the cloves into medicines. A pyramid-builder carved into his monument the amount of garlic consumed by his work crews.

This pungent root is one of humanity's earliest healers, and it is now being rediscovered by medical scientists who long consigned it to the kitchen. In the past 20 years more than 1,000 articles have been published on the remarkable healing qualities of garlic plants.

Garlic is used to fight fever, stomach ache, parasites, dysentery and toxemia. What's in this lowly root that can heal all these ailments?

Scientists' first answer was allicin - a substance excreted from the garlic bulb when it is squeezed or bruised. Allicin is a natural antibiotic. It kills bacteria, fungi and intestinal parasites. But that's not all!

Garlic also contains 32 sulphur compounds, 17 amino acids, selenium, magnesium, potassium, germanium, copper, iron, zinc, vitamins A, B1 and C. First, let's look at the sulphur:

SULPHUR AND CANCER

The Japanese have known for centuries about the healing effects of sulphur. To this day, those suffering from a wide array of ailments flock to "Shira Ne San" or "White Root Mountain" in northern Japan. They dip themselves into a natural hot spring halfway up the mountain, where the sulfuric content and heat is supposed to cure just about anything.

Large amounts of sulphur naturally occur in garlic. The compounds stop cancer-producing cells from forming, and stops the enzymes that encourage metastasis - the spread of cancer.

Diallyl sulfide (DAS), has been shown to stop stomach and lung cancers in mice. Though scientists aren't sure how the compound works, they found a significant increase in detoxifying enzymes in the stomachs of mice given DAS in garlic form. The more garlic they were fed, the more of these cancer-fighting enzymes were found.

Another study found that garlic slows the growth of tumor cells while it speeds the growth of healthy tissue. In a review of 30 nutritional studies, doctors found that garlic and onion consumption plays a significant role in the reduced number of cancer deaths.

A GARLIC CONGRESS

In 1990, the First World Congress on the Health Significance of Garlic and Garlic Constituents was held in Washington, DC. It was sponsored by Pennsylvania State University, the US Department of Agriculture and an international garlic producer. Some of the healing discoveries shared at the symposium were as follows:

Aged garlic acts as a natural shield against radiation damage. Rats and rabbits were exposed to cobalt-60 gamma rays. Those treated before exposure with garlic had higher white blood counts, less leakage of enzymes into the blood stream and lower death rates. White blood cells are a natural component of a healthy immune system. Doctors concluded that garlic may help maximize the body's immunity.

Penn State researchers found that aged garlic extract powder protects against breast cancer in rats. A group of rats was exposed to breast cancer - half of them were pretreated with garlic supplements; the others were fed a normal diet. Of the garlic group, 35 percent developed breast cancer. But 90 percent of the untreated group developed the disease. The scientists said the garlic prevents cancer-causing substances from binding to the genetic material in the breast tissue cells, thus preventing formation of tumors.

Doctors at UCLA studied the effect of aged garlic on skin cancer. They found garlic stopped cancer growth in 50 percent of the laboratory samples they studied. Indeed, after applying garlic to melanoma cells, the cancerous tissue appeared normal!

Garlic is now under study at the National Cancer Institute, the US Department of Agriculture and Loma Linda University. Scientists there hope to understand soon how garlic enhances the immune system, stops cancer growth and lowers blood pressure.

A statement issued after the World Congress warned consumers of false advertisements issued by garlic producers anxious to cash in on the herb's healing properties. These usually claim high concentrations of allicin, and recommend large doses to affect cures. However, garlic is classified by Chinese herbalists as moderately toxic - too much can cause stomach cramping and an unpleasant buildup of intestinal gas. Let the buyer beware.

TOMATOES, TOO, ARE GOOD FOR YOU

The tomato is a major source of lycopene, a potent antioxidant. Tomatoes are linked to a lowered incidence of bladder cancer, and are at the top of the "best vegetables" list released by the FDA Consumer magazine.

WE CAN HEAL OURSELVES

Our bodies must be nutritionally rich, overflowing with natural enzymes that feed on dangerous free radicals. We need not spend hundreds of dollars on expensive prescriptions or special diet foods - these natural cancer-fighters are as close as the produce section of the grocery store or our backyard gardens.

Chapter V

The Importance of Dietary Fats

The Essential Fatty Acids vs The Destructive Fats

Both the National Cancer Society and the American Heart Association have stated that, in general, the average daily fat consumption of the American people is excessive. These two organizations, both dedicated to improving the health of the nation, have issued dietary guidelines which strongly suggest that we can reduce our risk of developing cancer (and the other degenerative diseases) simply by trimming (at least) 10 percent of the fat from our daily menus and eating lean.

On the surface of it, this seems to be an easy guideline to observe. It's really not difficult for the family cook to skim off the fat that rises to the top of the pot when making soups, stews, and gravies. A fish sauced with lemon and herbs is even more delicious than a greasy hamburger, and a lot healthier. Every supermarket in the country carries well-known and heavily advertised name brands of margarines and vegetable oils that proudly claim to be free of the saturated fats that promote harmful blood cholesterol levels. Every refrigerator case in every supermarket in every locale holds a vast selection of low-fat dairy products. Even salad dressings and mayonnaises especially processed to be low in fat are now readily available.

But — *and it's a big but* — just how healthy are these commercially processed fats and oils? Because medical researchers and scientists all over the world have found that the excessive consumption of dietary fats can be dangerous to our health, we decided to do some serious in-depth digging to find out the *real* story behind the brief dietary guidelines suggesting a reduction in fats which have been issued in recent years.

FATS & OILS IN HISTORY

Mankind has used the natural fats for both food and other purposes since prehistoric times. There is evidence showing that the early Egyptians made use of olive oil in flavoring, preparing, and preserving foodstuffs, as well as using it as a lubricant in moving the immense building blocks of the ancient pyramids. They also made a very efficient axle grease from fat and lime. As far back as 1400 BC, Homer tells us that oil was an aid to the weaver. Pliny mentions both hard and soft soaps, made with wood ashes and fats. In Biblical times, olive oil was so highly regarded that it was used in preparing offerings to the Lord (Leviticus 2:1), and for holy annointings (Exodus 30:22), as well as gracing the family table as a worthy staple of life.

THE OIL PROCESSING INDUSTRY — The industry as we know it has been growing by leaps and bounds for over fifty years. However, medical detectives and scientists have made some startling discoveries in the past two decades about the way fat metabolism works (or doesn't work) in the body. Perhaps if we had known fifty years ago what we know *now* about the ways in which chemically altered fats lead irrevocably to a host of degenerative diseases, the government might have taken a different position on these products. According to reliable sources, the methods used by the commercial oil industry to manufacture dietary fats are subject to 'periodic' review and re-evaluation by the Food & Drug Administration. In light of the growing masses of clinical research about the harmful effects of excessive fat intake, perhaps it's time to call for the FDA to exercise their prerogatives and do a thorough review of industry manufacturing methods in order to update their records.

In the so-called civilized societies, the increased incidence of the degenerative diseases (cancer, cardiovascular disease, diabetes, multiple sclerosis, liver and kidney problems) have paralleled the increased consumption of unnatural chemically altered fats. That may be a bold statement, but it's easily documented. A whopping 57 percent of our dietary fat consumption now comes from commercially processed fats and oils, such as margarine, shortening, salad, and cooking oils. At the turn of the century, cancer claimed the life of one person in every thirty, but today it kills one in five. One hundred years ago, heart disease took one person in every seven. The cardiovascular toll is now one person in every two.

DESTRUCTIVE 'INDUSTRIAL STRENGTH' FATS

You may find it hard to believe what the commercial oil industry does with some perfectly natural seeds before you find the finished products (margarine, cooking and salad oils, shortening) on the shelves of your neighborhood grocery stores. Here's what happens:

'COLD-PRESSED' — After the seeds are cleaned, they are mechanically crushed and subjected to fierce temperatures (the average is around 248 degrees F.) in order to break down the cell walls, thereby making the extraction of the oil easier. Because the vital live enzymes cannot survive temperatures much over 110 degrees F., it's already too late to save the enzymes, but we're just beginning. Next, the unappetizing dead mash of cooked seeds is forced through a giant press that works very much like an old-fashioned kitchen meat grinder. The difference is that this press exerts tremendous pressure (up to several tons per square inch). As the screw inexorably turns, the seeds are crushed and forced against the press head. This friction generates more heat (up to 203 degrees F.). This combination of friction-generated heat and press-crushing forces the seed to give up its oil.

If the processing stops here, these oils are allowed to be sold (usually in health-food stores at a premium price) as 'cold-pressed,' 'natural,' 'crude,' or 'unrefined.' Most authorities agree that the temperatures generated in the processing are high

93

enough to cause deterioration of the essential fatty acids. As hard as it may be to believe, these 'cold-pressed' oils are the highest quality currently available from U.S. manufacturers.

'UNREFINED OIL' — Another favored method of extraction consists of using a chemical solvent to leach the oil from seeds. After being crushed and cooked, the seeds are then mechanically ground and processed with a chemical solvent at temperatures of up to 149 degrees F. (One popular solvent is *hexane,* manufactured from petroleum). You should know that the solvent is reclaimed after batches of seeds have been processed and is reused many times. Oils extracted with chemicals are unavoidably tainted with traces of these chemicals. Very often, chemically extracted oils are mixed with 'cold-pressed' oils. These oils find their way to stores and are marketed as 'unrefined oils.'

YOU ASKED FOR IT

Consumers have been brain-washed into believing that their salad and cooking oils should be clear, free-pouring at any temperature, odorless, and tasteless. Without commercial processing, natural oils offer the delicate taste characteristic of the seeds from which they came. They range in color from a pale yellow to gold to amber to almost red. Their different aromas are as distinctive as their different tastes. If you put them in the refrigerator, they become cloudy and their viscosity changes. In other words, they become somewhat heavier and thicker.

THE REFINING PROCESS — The first step in refining the oil, called degumming, is to remove most of the remaining phosphatides, essential for life. Lecithin (an important unsaturated fatty acid) is taken out. All the complex carbohydrates, some elements similar to proteins, and the gums are removed. The chlorophyll, calcium, magnesium, iron, and copper (health-promoting minerals) are also refined out.

Second, some caustic corrosive chemicals, such as sodium hydroxide (better known as Draino), or a mixture of sodium hydroxide and sodium carbonate, are dumped into the oil. The

94

nasty mess is then mechanically agitated at a temperature of approximately 167 degrees F. The remaining free fatty acids combine with the caustic chemicals to form easily removed 'soaps.' Just about all that's left of the remaining minerals, protein-like elements, and phospholipids (fats with phosphorous and nitrogen), are eliminated during this stage of the 'refining' process. But the oil may be yellowish or reddish in color, still hanging on to a little of its identity in the form of pigments.

The third step consists of bleaching out the natural pigments to provide you with that colorless oil you've been taught to expect. Beta-carotene (a documented cancer-preventive) and chlorophyll, along with the last traces of the fatty acids, are filtered out, usually with acid-based clays, at temperatures of up to 230 degrees F. The essential fatty acids still present are further chemically damaged and may form toxic peroxides.

Deodorizing is the fourth step in the refining process. You couldn't possibly recognize the seed source of the oil at this point. The delicate flavor and scent that Mother Nature puts into her seeds has been replaced by unappetizing chemical odors and tastes. Taking out the bad taste and smell is accomplished by the use of a steam distilling process at extremely high temperatures (up to 518 degrees F.) for a period lasting as long as an hour. Thankfully, the dangerous peroxides and toxins produced in the previous step are removed, along with some of the pesticide residue. But the deodorizing process also eliminates the Vitamin E. *And,* of immense concern to all of us, the essential fatty acids have been transformed into something completely foreign to the human body.

The tortured oil must undergo yet another couple of steps before you buy it and take it home. Because the natural antioxidants (beta-carotene and Vitamin E) have been removed from the oil in the 'refining process,' synthetic chemical antioxidants are pumped in to lengthen the shelf life and a 'defoamer' is also added. And, because some of us refrigerate our salad and cooking oils, it is usually subjected to a process known in the industry as 'winterization.' The oil is artifically cooled and filtered yet again to insure that it remains clear

95

under refrigeration. (This is the 'polyunsaturated oil' that is commonly added to commercial baby-formulas to provide 'essential fatty acids.')

The end result is an oil that is clear, odorless, tasteless, and indistinguishable from any other oil manufactured in the same manner. Unless the label tells you, there's absolutely no way to tell what the original seed source might have been. With all the vitamins and minerals eliminated, and the essential fatty acid molecules chemically altered, that oil on your supermarket shelves is a highly questionable food item.

ADDING INSULT TO INJURY

THE HYDROGENATION PROCESS — Even if the industry started with a completely natural oil (and they don't, they start with a chemically altered oil), the hydrogenation process destroys all nutritional value. Hydrogenating the oil consists of completely saturating all of the fatty acids with hydrogen. Hydrogenation is accomplished under pressure by using temperatures of up to 410 degrees F. in the company of a metal catalyst (nickel, platinum, copper) for as long as eight hours. Because the final product is a completely inert (dead) substance, it doesn't spoil and can be heated for (or in) cooking without becoming dangerously toxic. But it contains chemically altered bits of fatty acids, some of which may be harmful, and traces of the metal catalyst.

PARTIAL HYDROGENATION — By controlling the length of the hydrogenation process, a liquid oil can be transformed into a solid or semi-solid mass of fat. When the desired degree of hardness is attained, the hydrogenation process is stopped. Margarines and solid shortenings are manufactured with partially hydrogenated oils. Although logically you might not think so, *partially* hydrogenated products are actually more dangerous to your health than *fully* hydrogenated products. Here's why:

The molecules in the oil being bombarded with hydrogen become saturated (hydrogenated) erratically, leaving behind a proliferation of strangely altered substances when the process is halted. Many of these chemically alien elements are

96

identified as being harmful because they interfere with the body's normal metabolism. Many others have not been scientifically researched and we just don't know what dangers they may pose when ingested.

MARGARINE — The Encyclopedia Britannica tells us that French chemist Hippolyte Mege-Mouries invented 'artificial butter' back in 1869. Mege-Mouries won the prize offered by Napoleon, who wanted a cheap fat to feed his soldiers and sailors, with his combination of skim milk and suet (melted beef fat). Although this disagreeable early butter substitute tasted just as awful as it sounds, it caught on. Mege-Mouries secured a patent for his process in the United States in 1873 and the industry as we know it today began.

As time passed, the animal fats used in the beginning gave way to imported vegetable fats, usually cottonseed, soybean, peanut, and corn oils, and the product became more palatable. The early manufacture of margarine was subject to strong restrictive legislation in the U.S. because both the butter producers and the nation's farmers feared for their livelihood. However, during the 1930s, U.S. farmers began supplying cottonseed and soybeans and the fledgling 'artificial butter' industry was on its way. As recently as the World War II years, margarine was sold uncolored. The white block, looking like a brick of shortening, came with a packet of powdered yellow-orange dye which the housewife had to blend in, usually by squeezing it through the softened mass with her hands.

No matter what seed oil the margarine manufacturer starts with, and usually the cheapest source is used, the essential fatty acids present to start with are either destroyed or changed in the hydrogenation process into chemically altered substances. The essential fatty acids that remain fight with the carbon fatty acids and reduce the nutritional value of the essentials still further. Add to this the fact that the minerals and vitamins the body needs for efficient metabolism of fats were ,refined' out and you have a nearly indigestible fat.

A very efficient advertising campaign has led us to believe that margarine is good for us because it's made with polyunsaturated fats. We equate polyunsaturates with good health because we know that the essential fatty acids are polyun-saturates. But what they don't tell us is that the polyunsaturates in margarine are *not* the essential fatty acids the body cries out for, but chemically altered alien fats. It is true that margarine contains no cholesterol, but the presence of so many chemicals completely alien to the body cancels out that small advantage. Remember, there is a lot of evidence showing that these chemically altered fats are strongly implicated in the degenerative diseases.

HOW MUCH IS TOO MUCH? — A lot of very authoritative medical scientists hold the position that the body reacts adversely to even a smidgin of a chemically altered alien substance. The cumulative effects of regularly consuming a diet high in chemically altered fats are devastating.

Studies show that hard margarines contain an average of over 30 percent chemically altered fatty acids. (Some brands register a whopping 60 percent.) Soft margarines (and diet margarines) contain an average of close to 20 percent chemically altered fatty acids. The measureable *essential* fatty acids present in margarines are virtually zero — less than 5 percent in all brands tested.

Hard vegetable shortenings tallied an average of 20 percent chemically altered fatty acids, with some brands containing close to 40 percent. Vegetable salad oils contain nearly 15 percent chemically altered fatty acids.

Commercially made baked goods average nearly 35 percent chemically altered fatty acids. Candies contain close to 40 percent chemically altered fatty acids. Even that old standby, peanut butter, contains varying amounts of chemically altered fatty acids. I hate to tell you about french fries (up to 40 percent) and potato chips (another 40 percent).

IS BUTTER BETTER? — Cattle, goats, and sheep have been kept by man for the production of milk and milk products for as long as history has been recorded, and probably even earlier than that. As far back as 1200 BC, Hindu writings mention the use of butter as food. The early Europeans used butter, not as a food, but as a remedy for skin injuries and sore eyes. It was also widely used as a hair oil and as fuel for lamps.

Is butter better than margarine? Well, it is certainly natural and certainly *tastes* better. Unfortunately, of the 500 fatty acids which have been identified in butter, only a very small percentage are the essentials (linoleic acid 2%, linolenic acid, trace). Over 65 percent of butter's fatty acid content requires the same elements for metabolism as the essentials. If the non-essential fatty acids outnumber the essentials, it's easy to understand that the non-essentials will win the metabolic battle. Butter also contains a small (less than 5 percent) amount of chemically altered fatty acids. Unlike the chemically processed fats and oil discussed earlier, these altered fats are produced in the cow itself and are not a serious health risk.

Butter does contain about 1 gram of cholesterol in every pound. We're going to tell you the truth about cholesterol, required by every cell in the body, a little later in this chapter. For now, what you should remember is that the average diet is sadly lacking in the elements (essential fatty acids, certain vitamins and minerals) needed to process cholesterol efficiently. The natural diet consumed by our ancestors had these elements in abundance.

Another drawback is that our modern-day butter also registers the presence of unwanted pesticides and antibiotics. The cows feed on grasses and grains that are pesticide-treated. Antibiotics are routinely given to the animals themselves and commercially manufactured feed is treated with antibiotics. The target is harmful disease-promoting bacteria, which are destroyed by the antibiotic treatment. But some friendly bacteria have developed resistance to the drugs. With good reason, researchers fear that the resistance factor can cross over to the dangerous bacteria, making them less susceptible to antibiotics.

In favor of butter, we must point out that it can be used in and for all types of cooking without breaking down into dangerous toxins. It is stable in the presence of light, heat, and oxygen. The relatively small percentage of naturally-occurring altered fatty acids is not a threat to health, but you can't depend on butter for your supply of essential fatty acids. Butter is easy to digest and the cholesterol content is not harmful, as long as your diet contains the elements necessary for the efficient metabolism of fat. However, even this natural dietary fat can create problems when consumed in excess. To sum it all up, butter *is* better for you, unless you're a glutton about it.

It's important to remember that fatty acids are essential to life. They play a vital part in the functioning of the entire body. It's therefore very important to seek out and incorporate good sources of the right kind of fatty acids into your daily diet. The following diagram illustrates the relationships of polyunsaturated dietary fatty acids and their influence on human diseases.

Presence of Polyunsaturated Fatty Acids in Various Oils and Their Influence on Human Diseases.

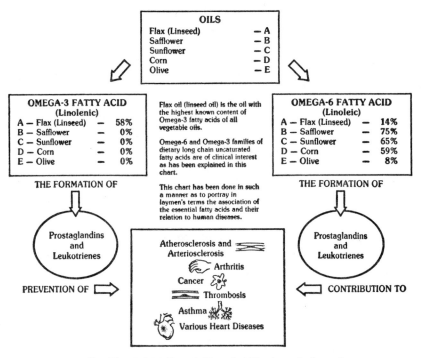

Flax oil (linseed oil) is the best seed oil for people with fatty degeneration, because the oil contains the largest amount of the most strongly dispersing essential fatty acid, the three times unsaturated linolenic acid (LNA = linolenic acid = Omega-3).

LNA helps to disperse from our tissues deposits of the saturated fatty acids and cholesterol, which like to aggregate and which make platelets sticky. (Platelets play an important role in blood coagulation and blood thrombus formation.) The oil has to be fresh, and not exposed to light, oxygen, and heat, because these three agents destroy the essential fatty acids very rapidly. Flax oil (linseed oil) should be *unrefined*,

*From "Fats and Oils — The Complete Guide to Fats and Oils in Health and Nutrition," by Udo Erasmus, Alive Books, Vancouver, B. C.

THE MYSTIQUE OF CHOLESTEROL — There are so many misconceptions and half-truths surrounding the workings of cholesterol in the human body that it seems like a good idea to remind you that cholesterol is required by every cell in the body *and* is the raw material from which the body produces bile acids, certain hormones, and provitamin D3. Simply eliminating cholesterol from the diet doesn't work. The body can manufacture up to about 1½ grams of cholesterol every day, and does, if it isn't supplied in the diet. It really isn't the level of cholesterol in the blood that creates health problems, it's whether the body has the elements it needs to process it properly.

THE IMPORTANT FATS

Because we're already on the subject of cholesterol, it seems appropriate to again explain the relationship between the essential fatty acids and cholesterol here. Cholesterol is dissolved and held in suspension in a free-flowing liquid state in the blood in the presence of adequate essential fatty acids. Because the melting point of cholesterol is 300 degrees F., it is deposited on arterial walls as an insoluble substance at the normal body temperature of 98.6 degrees F. With the fatty acid *lecithin* present, the melting point of cholesterol is reduced to 180 degrees F., still insoluble at body temperature. But when the essential fatty acids *linoleic* and *linolenic* are in sufficient supply, the melting point of cholesterol comes down to 32 degrees F., well below normal body temperature. In a liquid state, cholesterol cannot end up as harmful arterial plaque and does not promote the degenerative diseases.

FISH OIL — There's been a lot written lately about the omega-3 fatty acids (*eicosapentaenoic acid* (EPA) and *docosahexaenoic acid* (DHA) present in the arterial-cleansing fish oils. The fact that Eskimos and the Scandinavian peoples eat a lot of cold-water fish (rich sources of EPA and DHA) and enjoy a very low incidence of degenerative disease led researchers to study the workings of these two highly unsaturated fatty acids in the body. It was determined that EPA and DHA help lower the melting point of the saturated fats, thus keeping them from attaching themselves to arterial walls.

The important polyunsaturated fatty acids of marine origin enter the human food chain via a simple process. They are formed naturally in underwater plants and organisms, such as phytoplankton and algae. Many fish feed on these sea creatures and other larger fish, in turn, feed on them. As these elements are incorporated into the flesh of marine life, the fatty acids are welcomed into their lipid structure. The fish oils that are important to human life are present in their purest and most concentrated form in the fish that swim in the cold oceans of the world. Science says that it is the low temperature of this environment which dictates that their fatty acids should be of the highly unsaturated type.

However, the oils of many marine species contain toxic fatty acids which are harmful to humans. Cetoleic acid, shown to foster fatty degeneration of the heart, is present in herring oil, cod liver oil, and the oils of menhaden and anchovetta. And warm-water species and lean low-fat fish may be tasty and nutritious, but don't provide the important omega-3 fatty acids that protect against heart disease and cancer.

The world's leading authority on the omega-3 fatty acids present in marine oils is acknowledged to be the brilliant Danish professor, J. Dyerberg, M.D., Ph.D. Dr. Dyerberg heads the Department of Clinical Chemistry at the Aalborg Hospital (Aalborg, Denmark) and is responsible for a number of landmark papers on the effects of the polyunsaturated fatty acids, particularly in the treatment and prevention of atherosclerosis.

Dr. Dyerberg has an explanation for the failure of most nutritional authorities to recommend the daily intake of marine oils until recently. He says, "Fish oils were originally not mentioned in most dietary guidelines to lower serum cholesterol and prevent atherosclerosis. One reason for this might be that the populations most concerned with preventing atherosclerotic diseases do not readily accept and enjoy eating seafood. Another reason is that the long-chain polyunsaturated fats have low melting points and are easily oxidized. These qualities create problems in the manufacture of margarine and shortening. Reports published in the 1950s and 1960s indicating that fish oil may lower blood cholesterol even more than vegetable oil had no major impact on early dietary recommendations. The first real breakthrough concerning dietary fats occurred with the report of the clinical effects on coronary atherosclerosis of a diet rich in seafood."

In conjunction with H. O. Bang, it was Dr. Dyerberg who initiated the dietary studies of the Greenland Eskimos in the late 1970s. This report was published in 1981 in *Acta Scandanavia* Vol. 210: 245-248. Building on earlier research, the scientists uncovered the reason for the very low incidence of cardiovascular disease in Eskimo society. Although the population ate a very high fat diet (known to promote heart disease) of whale, seal, and walrus meat, they universally consumed a lot of cold-water fish as well.

After expanding his study to include Greenlanders, Dr. Dyerberg explains, "Statistics from Greenland show a low mortality rate from ischemic heart disease (atherosclerosis) with no sex difference. From 45 to 64 years of age, 25 out of 277 male deaths (9 percent) and 13 out of 178 female deaths (7 percent), or 38 out of 455 deaths (8.4 percent) in both sexes were recorded in a 5-year period within a population of approximately 50,000. In the community of 2000 inhabitants which we studied, which had a hospital with ECG facilities, 10 years of medical records did not include a single death from ischemic heart disease."

Within the last few decades, cardiovascular disease has risen steadily in Japan. As the Japanese people have embraced western dietary preferences in place of their traditionally high consumption of fish, the rate of death from cardiovascular disease has kept pace. As they have dropped fish from the menu and patronize McDonald's instead, the Japanese no longer enjoy their previous immunity from heart disease. Western disease patterns are now apparent in the population of Japan.

Most of us would not find a daily diet of fish palatable. It would be difficult indeed for the typical American to choke down the amount of fish that gives the Eskimos their seeming immunity to heart disease. However, a Dutch scientist by the name of D. Kromhout recognized the problems such a diet would pose to the western world and had a study already in progress to determine exactly what quantity of fish a person would have to eat to enjoy its protective effect. The results of Kromhout's study were published in the *New England Journal of Medicine* in 1985. Here's what he found:

In order to calculate the relationship between the measured intake of fish and coronary mortality, Kromhout selectively chose a group of 852 middle-aged men whose dietary habits could be determined for the 20-year period of the study. He assigned risk factors according to the amount of fish normally consumed. Men who disliked fish and never ate it at all were found to have a risk factor of 1.0. Those men eating from 1 to 14 grams of fish had a risk factor of 0.64; those consuming 15 to 29 grams had a risk factor of 0.56; and those eating 30 to 144 grams of fish every day had a risk factor of 0.36. After reviewing Kromhout's data, Dr. Dyerberg noted, "The interesting observation made by Kromhout is the inverse relationship between a relatively low level of fish intake and coronary heart disease. This finding makes nutritional advice based on the seafood hypothesis much easier to give and accept, compared to that based on data from Greenland and Japan which describe fish intakes that are unrealistically high for many people."

HEART HEALTH & MUCH MORE — Both EPA and DHA are present in the most important and active organs and tissues of the body, including the brain cells, the nervous system, and the sex glands. The omega-3 fatty acids play a very important part in regulating the chemical balance of the body and assist in normalizing the coagulation factor of the blood. In impressive double-blind clinical studies, fish oil has been shown to possess remarkable arterial-cleansing ability. It has reduced cholesterol and triglyceride levels, markedly lowered dangerously high blood pressure, eased the pain of rheumatoid arthritis, worked against migraines, and has even shown protective effects against cancer. The researchers are onto something big. Here's what they're saying now:

Both the American Heart Association and the American Cancer Society have published research showing that the American diet is both excessively high in the wrong kinds of fats and woefully deficient in the right kinds of fats. Health experts around the world have documented the health problems arising as a result of consuming too much fat. Physicians routinely monitor cholesterol and triglyceride levels to determine those at high risk of suffering a heart attack.

Heart Disease: Cardiologists and doctors all over the world are now prescribing fish oils as a proven therapeutic measure for those with dangerously high cholesterol and triglyceride readings. In clinical tests, omega-3 fish oils were shown to almost miraculously lower harmful blood fats, while increasing beneficial blood fats that protect against heart disease.

In the *New England Journal of Medicine,* Dr. Michael Davidson of St. Luke's Medical Center reported on a study of patients taking fish oil capsules which showed spectacular results. Overall cholesterol levels dropped 24% and triglyceride levels fell 48%. Dr. Davidson pointed out that simply taking fish oil capsules cut the risk of suffering a fatal heart attack by 50% for these patients.

Cancer: Germany's premiere biochemist, Dr. Johanna Budwig favors a nutritional approach to the treatment of cancer. As an important part of the diet, she feeds her cancer patients freshly caught rainbow trout, a good source of the omega-3 fatty acids. Dr. Budwig has demonstrated the incredible tumor-dissolving effects of EPA, DHA, linolenic and linoleic acids in her practice and is noted for her seemingly miraculous cures of terminal cancer patients, extensively detailed in the following chapter (Chapter 6).

Studies indicate that a high-fat diet can foster cancer. But recent studies coming from Dr. Michael Pariza of the University of Wisconsin are beginning to alter scientific thinking. Dr. Pariza showed that 75 percent of lab animals fed a high-fat/HIGH-CALORIE diet got cancer, but only a tiny 7 percent of the animals fed a high-fat/LOW-CALORIE diet developed tumors. It has long been known that obesity adds to the risk of cancer. Cutting fat from the diet is an efficient way to lose pounds, but cutting calories may be more effective.

New research shows that the omega-3 fatty acids actually suppress some cancer-promoting substances. Rutgers University researcher Dr. Rashida A. Karmali says early indications are that omega-3 may protect against breast and prostate cancer. Dr. Karmali says, "Animals given fish oil had a significantly lower rate of cancers when exposed to cancer-causing agents or when they received transplanted tumors." Other scientists have reported similar findings against colon and lung cancers.

Dr. William E. Connor, Oregon Health Sciences University: "There is more and more evidence indicating that omega-3 fatty acids have a fundamental role in human health, both as a necessary nutrient and to prevent certain diseases occurring as a result of a chemical imbalance."

Arthritis: Until now, medical science held out no real hope of curing arthritis. The treatment of choice consists mainly of giving anti-inflammatory drugs, such as aspirin, to reduce pain and swelling. British researchers recently discovered that the herb Feverfew works better than aspirin, has no harmful side effects, and the pain relieving anti-inflammatory benefits of Feverfew actually last longer.

Because both Feverfew and fish oils are natural food substances with no known harmful side effects, some authorities believe that a combination of the two could spell real relief for arthritics.

Another useful, completely natural adjunct to the treatment of arthritis are the omega-3 fatty acids. Joel M. Kremer, M.D. of Albany Medical College explains that a group of eicosanoids called leukotrienes have been identified as a possible cause of the pain and inflamed joints of rheumatoid arthritis. When the omega-3 fatty acids in fish oil are supplemented in the diet, the chemical composition of the leukotrienes becomes almost magically less inflammatory.

In a recent 12-week long double-blind study of arthritis patients, Dr. Kremer found that patients given 1.8 grams of a concentrated fish oil supplement reported greatly reduced pain and swelling. Calling the results "very encouraging," Dr. Kremer noted that the control patients in the study who were given an inert substance instead of fish oil showed no improvement.

Psoriasis: Because leukotrienes are believed to be responsible for the inflammation and scaling of severe psoriasis, some scientists are calling fish oil a possible treatment for this disfiguring skin disease. As reported in the *Annals of Allergy,* early British and U.S. studies report that fish oil supplements brought welcome relief to some (but not all) psoriasis sufferers.

Reducing Rejection: More good news from the *Journal of Surgical Research* reveals that a diet high in the omega-3 fatty acids lowers the risk of rejection when surgical tissue grafts are necessary. After noting this effect in laboratory animals, the scientists theorized that fish oil supplements work by altering the clotting factor of blood platelets, thereby reducing the body's rejection response to a foreign graft.

Overall: Dr. William Lands, Chief of Biological Chemistry, University of Illinois states: "We now understand the disease process much better and see that there is a dietary linkage. The potential for major improvements in health, not necessarily from a therapeutic point of view, but from a preventive medicine point of view, are really tremendous."

FISH OIL SUPPLEMENTS FLOOD THE MARKET — Certain fresh and salt water fish from icy cold northern waters have been determined to be excellent sources of EPA and DHA. In order of their importance, they are salmon, sardines, mackerel trout, and eel. The omega-3 content of fresh salmon has been measured as between 18.9 percent and 31.4 percent of its total fat content. Lean low-fat fish, including pike, carp, and haddock, also contain EPA and DHA, but in minute quantities. The best source of the omega-3 fatty acids is salmon, but salmon is very expensive. Most of us wouldn't find it practical or even particularly pleasant to eat salmon every day. The easy way to add the protective effects of these wonder-working fatty acids to your daily diet appears to be as simple as selecting a good dietary supplement.

As more and more reports of the wonders of the omega-3 fatty acids have been picked up from the medical journals and trumpeted from the housetops, more and more manufacturers have come out with fish oil supplements. Unless you have considerable knowledge, choosing the right fish oil dietary supplement can be risky. For instance, if the fish oil in your capsule has been obtained from salmon (or trout) raised on a fish farm, the quality of the oil is inferior. The elements essential to the production of the omega-3 fatty acids in the fish are put in commercial fish foods, but deteriorate rapidly. Fish raised in a shallow tank or pond, in contrast to those swimming free and feeding on fresh, live marine animals and the rich vegetation of the sea, just cannot be considered a good source of EPA and DHA.

Another important point to consider when selecting a fish oil dietary supplement has to be the method of manufacture. EPA and DHA (and linolenic acid) are destroyed by light, air, and heat. These super-sensitive fatty acids must be handled delicately. Capsules must be filled quickly under stringent manufacturing procedures which insure that light, air, and heat are excluded. And the capsule shell must be opaque and dense enough to protect the precious contents from deterioration.

After doing an in-depth investigation of the fish oil products currently available, we have found what we believe to be the best fish oil supplement available anywhere. We think it's important to bring this little-known fish oil supplement to your attention.

Salmon Oil (from Scandinavia), is a concentrated source of the important omega-3 fatty acids derived ONLY from salmon caught in the crystal-clear and pristine unpolluted waters off the Norwegian coast. Unlike many of the newly popular fish oil supplements, *Salmon Oil* is just that — pure salmon oil — not a conglomeration of mixed fish oils. This very special product has 1000 mg of salmon oil, each contains 120 mg EPA and 80 mg of DHA in each pure capsule. No sugar, starch, artificial flavors or colors, chemical preservatives, yeast or sodium are added. You get pure deodorized salmon oil rich in omega-3 — and nothing else.

ONE FINAL OBSERVATION — Citing the work of German biochemist H. J. Mest ("The Influence of Linseed Oil Diet on Fatty Acid Pattern in Phospholipids & Thromboxane Formation in Platelets in Man," published in *Klin Wochenschr* in 1983), P.V. Johnston, Ph.D., of the University of Illinois (Urbana, Illinois), points out that Mest demonstrated an increase in the EPA and DHA content of serum phospholipids after several weeks of linseed oil supplementation.

Dr. Johnston says, "After four weeks, EPA was elevated 150 percent and DHA by 70 percent over initial levels." What this means is to you and me is that a *healthy* body can manufacture both EPA and DHA from linoleic acid, so they are not on the very exclusive list of essential fatty acids either. The problem is that few of us are housed in a truly healthy body working at optimum efficiency, so our production of EPA and DHA is inhibited. Let's tag EPA and DHA as very important fatty acids. *Arachidonic acid* is another important fatty acid, but most scientists agree that the body can produce arachidonic from linoleic acid. Therefore, it is not one of the true essentials.

However, as in most things, there is an exception which proves the rule. Laboratory studies of rats (reported in *Nutrition Reviews,* September 1986) show that the brain accumulates DHA and arachidonic acid quickly between birth and 20 days of age. This store correlates with a period of intense brain cell division. Between 20 and 40 days after birth, the rats show a heavy concentration of the fatty acids associated with the production of *myelin,* a protective sheath which covers all nerve fibers.

In an important paper entitled, "Fatty Acids in the Brain & Retina: Evidence for Their Essentiality," researchers M. Neuringer, Ph.D. (Oregon Health Sciences University and Oregon Regional Primate Research Center) and W. E. Connor, M.D. (Professor of Medicine, chief of the Division of Endocrinology, Metabolism & Clinical Nutrition, Oregon Health Sciences University, Portland, Oregon) explain how this relates to humans. "In human development, DHA and arachidonic acid accumulate rapidly both before and after birth. During the last trimester of pregnancy, cerebral and cerebellar content of these fatty acids increases three to five times; similar percent increases occur again between birth and twelve weeks of age.

"In primate (monkey) and human fetuses, levels of DHA and arachidonic acid are higher in the fetal blood than in maternal blood, whereas the opposite is true for their precursors, linolenic and linoleic acids. Selective incorporation mechanisms appear to exist to supply the fetal brain with the relatively high levels of DHA needed for normal development. After birth, newborn infants may be limited in their capacity to synthesize DHA and arachidonic acid from linolenic and linoleic acids and may be dependent on direct dietary sources. Human breast milk contains sufficient amounts of DHA and arachidonic acid to provide sufficient amounts for the developing brain. However, most synthetic human infant formulas provide no DHA or arachidonate. Infants fed these formulas have far less DHA in their blood fats than infants receiving human milk, even when ample linolenic acid is provided."

This is yet another bit of evidence showing that the mother who is able and nurses her child gives him a head start. A pregnant woman is well advised to make sure that her diet includes an adequate supply of these fatty acids, both while she is carrying the child and after delivery as well if she is planning to breastfeed her infant.

In the same paper, Drs. Neuringer and Connor point out that there is a growing body of evidence showing that EPA and DHA (of the n-3 group) should be classified as essential fatty acids on a par with linolenic acid (also an n-3 fatty acid), long known to be one of the true essentials. The scientists say that the n-3 fatty acids are important to the structure and function of membranes, particularly in the retina and central nervous system. Fish, shellfish, and marine mammals are a rich source of the n-3 fatty acids, including DHA, meaning that the body is not required to synthesize it.

In the body, high concentrations of DHA are present in the retina of the eye, the cerebral cortex of the brain, the testes and sperm. In fact, DHA makes up one-third of the fatty acid content of the cerebral cortex, explaining why fish has long been known as a 'brain food.' Because the body manufactures DHA from the essential fatty acids, the experts note that these high levels are automatically maintained by the body as long as dietary levels of the essential fatty acids are adequate. Studies show that deficiency symptoms can be reversed by supplying linolenic acid.

VEGETARIAN SOURCES OF OMEGA-3 FATTY ACIDS — *The New England Journal of Medicine* (Vol. 315, No. 13, 1986) recently published comments from A. P. Simopoulos, M.D. and N. Salem, Jr., Ph.D. (National Institute on Alcohol Abuse & Alcoholism) showing that *purslane* (Portulaca oleracea), a common garden herb which is better known as pigweed, is a good source of the omega-3 fatty acids. The authors point out that purslane is a common item on the menu in many Mediterranean countries which enjoy a low incidence of cancer and heart disease. They suggest that purslane could be a good source of the omega-3 fatty acids for vegetarians.

In the same issue, Michael A. Weiner, Ph.D. (Port Washington, New York) points out what he considers to be a drawback in the ingestion of fish oils. Dr. Weiner notes that, while dietary fish oils are prescribed for their antithrombotic and hypolipidemic effects, they contain a measure of cholesterol along with their healthy content of omega-3 fatty acids. However, because of the cholesterol-dissolving effect of EPA and DHA, many authorities discount this objection. Fortunately, for any of us who share Dr. Weiner's viewpoint, there are good plant sources of the omega-3 fatty acids. Dr. Weiner suggests that the botanicals might be a wiser choice for insuring that the important fatty acids are incorporated into the diet.

Because they are so important to your life and good health, it just makes good sense to plan meals which include the food sources of the important fatty acids. Before you do the family shopping, you might want to consult the following chart:

FOOD SOURCES & CELL DISTRIBUTION OF THE FATTY ACIDS

Fatty Acid	Food Sources	Cell Distribution
*Linolenic Acid** n-3	Crude Vegetable Oils Linseed, Soy, Walnut, Pumpkin	Component of all cells
*Linoleic Acid** n-6	Crude Vegetable Oils	Component of all cells
EPA (Eicosapentaenoic Acid) n-3	Fish & Shellfish (cold-water varieties)	Minor component of all cells
DHA (Docosahexaenoic Acid) n-3	Fish & Shellfish (cold-water varieties)	Major component of brain, retina (eye) testes, and sperm
Arachidonic Acid n-6	Liver, Brain, Meats	Component of most membranes
Oleic Acid n-9	Animal & Vegetable Fats	Component of many cells (white matter/myelin)
Docosapentaenoic Acid n-3	None	Low in normal cells (replaces DHA in EPA & linolenic deficiency)
Eicosatrienoic Acid n-9	None	Accumulates in total EPA deficiency syndrome

* Essential Fatty Acids

THE ESSENTIAL FATTY ACIDS

Both *linoleic acid* and *linolenic acid are essential to life.* This means that the body must have these fatty acids to survive, but cannot manufacture them from other elements in the diet. They must be supplied daily in the foods we eat. We have already pointed out one very important function of the essential fatty acids (linoleic and linolenic). They keep cholesterol in suspension, thereby preventing the buildup of the arterial plaque associated with cardiovascular disease and fatty degeneration.

Another important function of linoleic and linolenic acid is the transport of oxygen throughout the body. Every cell (blood, tissue, organ) requires oxygen for functioning. When the membranes surrounding and protecting each cell are pumped full of oxygen, harmful bacteria cannot enter. Bacteria and viruses don't grow in the presence of oxygen. The essentials are fashioned to absorb sunlight energy, immeasurably enhancing their ability to carry oxygen.

Because the essentials possess a slight negative electric charge, their molecules repel one another. It is this factor which moves toxins to the detoxifying systems of the body (intestinal tract, kidneys, liver, lungs, skin) where they can be eliminated. The electric charge they carry is also very important to the workings of the heart, nerves, and muscles. Acting like Mother Nature's 'pacemaker,' the essentials regulate the all-important beating of the heart.

Essential fatty acids control chromosomes during cell division and are necessary to the formation of new cell membranes after a cell has divided. Because we know that cancer cells are abnormal cells which grow and perpetuate themselves by division, it's easy to understand why the essential fatty acids are so important as both a preventive and treatment of any form of malignancy.

Overall cancer prevention requires a thorough knowledge of the metabolic pathways through which cancer spreads, the vascular supply of various parts of the body, the relationship of adjacent organs, as well as a clear understanding of both the normal and altered functions of the body.

DEFICIENCIES ARE SERIOUS — Many health authorities are beginning to realize that essential fatty acid deficiencies are widespread. It has been shown that the tissues and blood levels of the victims of the degenerative diseases are lacking in the essential fatty acids. In many cases, even if the important fatty acids are present, the elements the body needs to put them to work are missing. This is called a 'functional deficiency.'

When the diet is lacking in the essential fatty acids, serious health problems develop. The killers (cancer, heart disease,

113

and more) are fostered by an excessive intake of saturated fats (and chemically altered fats). Without the presence of the essential fatty acids, the killer diseases are given a very favorable environment. They thrive and grow, but we sicken and eventually die.

Other deficiency symptoms include liver and kidney degeneration, arthritis, circulatory problems, mood changes, vision complaints, hair loss, abnormal weakness, skin diseases, a lack of coordination, tingling in the extremities, inhibited growth, dryness of the mucous membranes (and glands), sterility in males, and miscarriages in females.

The September 1986 issue of *Nutrition Reviews* offers a clinical review of several cases of essential fatty acid (EFA) deficiency as observed in patients unable to take food by mouth and who were given fat-free TPN (total parenteral nutrition). A patient with short-bowel syndrome who was given fat-free TPN for 82 days showed all the classic symptoms of lineoleate deficiency. The article states: "Many of these patients had scaly skin (scleroderma), thrombocytopenia (an abnormal decrease in the number of blood platelets), and poor wound healing, accompanied by low levels of linoleic and arachidonic acid, and a high concentration of eicosatrienoic acid, strongly suggestive of linoleate deficiency."

When a female patient on fat-free TPN developed scleroderma, she was given 500 ml of plasma lipoproteins (fatty acids accompanied with red cell membranes) for a period of seven days. Her lipid values normalized promptly. In addition the visual disturbances which characterize an EFA deficiency were reversed simply by giving a linolenate-rich infusion.

Animal studies (National Academy of Science 1986) of monkeys showed that an EFA dietary deficiency produced retinal depletion of the n-3 fatty acids causing changes in vision. Pregnant female monkeys given a diet rich in safflower oil throughout their pregnancy, and to their infants after birth, exhibited sight abnormalities. An additional finding arising from this study indicates that the monkeys fed safflower oil had a reduced capacity for learning as well.

This important paper concludes with the suggestion that obstetricians and pediatricians should be aware that a linolenic deficiency of the pregnant mother is associated with visual and learning defects in the infant, especially if the infant's diet does not include sufficient EFA after birth.

The American Journal of Clinical Nutrition (Volume 44: September 1986) carried an article by E. M. Berry, M.D. MRCP and J. Hirsch, M.D. entitled "Does Dietary Linolenic Acid Influence Blood Pressure?" In this paper, Drs. Berry and Hirsch report on the long-term effects of polyunsaturated fats in the diet of 400 male subjects ranging in age from 20 to 78 years. They note that a mere one percent increase in dietary linolenic acid was associated with a corresponding healthy decrease in blood pressure.

This important work concludes, "Linolenic acid comprised only one-eighth the amount of linoleic acid, the major polyunsaturate in adipose (fatty) tissue and hence in the diet, yet it had a disproportionate association with BP (blood pressure). This may be related to its role as a precursor for the production of prostaglandins and/or other vasoregulators. Dietary manipulation with n-3 fatty acids may be helpful in the treatment and prevention of hypertension. Results suggest that linolenic acid, which is contained in linseed (flaxseed) oil, legumes, nuts, and citrus fruits, rather than linoleic acid may be the principle dietary polyunsaturated fatty acid related to blood pressure."

HOW MUCH IS ENOUGH? — Authoritative recommendations vary widely. How active you are physically, how stressed you are mentally, whether your daily diet is nutritionally correct, plus other factors personal to each of us, must all enter into an expert calculation of just how much of the essential fatty acids we individually need to consume every day. Most studies do agree, however, that males require up to three times as much of the essentials as females because of the differences in hormone production.

As a general rule of thumb, 9 to 30 grams daily (approximately 3 to 10 percent of the day's calories) of the essential fatty acids (linoleic and linolenic) seems to be about right for a normal person. Those of us who consume a diet high in saturated and chemically altered fats (and that includes the vast majority of the population), require the higher amount in order to rid the body of dangerous arterial plaque and gradually rebuild the cell and tissue damage caused by fatty degeneration.

Studies conducted with laboratory animals in which almost 30 percent of the day's calories were supplied in the form of linoleic acid resulted in no adverse changes in the animals over the long term, just as long as sufficient elements required for the processing of linoleic acid were also supplied. For efficient functioning, the body needs 1 part Vitamin E for every 1,500 parts linoleic acid. At the high end of the suggested daily allowance of essential fats (30 grams), around 50 I.U. of Vitamin E should be included in the diet. Other elements for efficient processing of the essential fatty acids include Vitamins A (or beta-carotene), C, B3, B6, and zinc.

FOOD SOURCES OF THE ESSENTIALS — As we have already discovered, the chemically altered fats present in common supermarket items like margarine, solid shortening, salad and cooking oils (and a lot of other commercially manufactured food products) are unhealthy in the extreme. You just cannot expect to get the essential fatty acids the body requires in these commercial products.

Be comforted. Mother Nature comes to the rescue with her delicious and very neatly packaged seeds and nuts. Remember, plants have the enzymes needed to manufacture the essential fatty acids, but man does not. It's no accident that the holy writings of many civilizations direct us to the plant kingdom, as in Ezekiel 47:12 —"...and the fruit thereof shall be for meat."

The very best and richest source of *both* the essential fatty acids (linoleic and linolenic) is *linseed oil*. (You're going to learn some incredible things about this oil a little later.) With 58 percent linolenic and close to 20 percent linoleic acid, linseed oil wins hands down, but there are a few other good natural sources as well. Pumpkin seed oil, soybean oil, and walnut oil contain both essentials, but are not as richly endowed as linseed oil. It is important that you know that these four sources provide the only oils which contain both essential fatty acids.

Olive oil, long a favorite of gourmets, contains no linolenic acid at all, and only 8 percent of its total fat content (20 percent) is present as linoleic acid. Also, despite what the manufacturers would like you to believe, corn oil contains not one trace of essential linolenic fatty acid. And, if you've been reading about safflower and evening primrose oil lately, you should know that they also contain only one of the essentials (linoleic acid), but offer no linolenic acid.

I almost hate to bring it up, but cottonseed, rapeseed, (commonly used in the commercial manufacture of vegetable oils, margarines, and solid shortenings) and peanut oil often contain toxins and toxic fatty acids. In addition, peanuts are easily contaminated by a toxic fungus that feeds on the damp legumes. (Strictly speaking, peanuts are not really nuts at all, but a member of the legume (bean pod) family.

NUTRITIONALLY PERFECT LINSEEDS

A nutritional analysis of this near-miraculous food reveals that mankind could very nearly sustain life on a diet consisting wholly of linseeds, probably more familiar to you as flax seed. Get ready for some surprising facts.

AMINO ACIDS — Linseed offers all of the essential amino acids, the ones the body requires but cannot manufacture. Replenishing the building blocks of life (proteins) is a daily requirement. If just one essential amino acid is missing from the diet, the resulting protein deficiency can lead to serious disease.

VITAMINS — Linseed is a rich source of the important fat-soluble Vitamins A, D, and E, plus B1, B2, and C (water-soluble). This should not come as a surprise. These are the vitamins the body needs to efficiently process the essential fatty acids. Even science is beginning to recognize that nature seldom slips up.

MINERALS — Linseed contains all the major minerals (potassium, phosphorus, magnesium, calcium, sulphur, iron,

117

zinc, sodium, chlorine), plus the important trace minerals (manganese, silicon, copper, fluorine, aluminum, nickel, cobalt, iodine, aolybdenum, chromium). If you recognize that selenium and vanadium are not listed, chalk it up to the fact that very likely the seeds were not tested for these only recently identified minerals.

FIBER — Linseed is considered an excellent source of fiber, required for healthy intestinal and colon functioning. Fiber assists in removing cholesterol, softens the stool, and relieves constipation. The experts point out that a diet high in fiber helps cleanse the toxins from the blood and liver and goes a long way toward improving the quality of life as we age.

MUCILAGE — The old-fashioned name for glue may have been mucilage, but that doesn't apply here. This gelatin-like substance reduces excess stomach acidity, soothes and lines the mucous membranes of the digestive and intestinal tracts (assuring a smooth trouble-free passage of stool), and helps move cholesterol along. Because it acts to regulate the glucose content of the blood, mucilage is believed useful to the diabetic as well.

LINSEED OIL IS NUTRITIONAL GOLD

Oil pressed from linseeds is incredibly rich in both essential fatty acids. It carries between 15 and 25 percent linoleic acid (twice unsaturated) and from 50 to 60 percent linolenic acid (three times unsaturated). As we have already examined, both are essential to the life processes and must be supplied in the diet. Linseed oil is also a very good source of beta-carotene (a precursor of Vitamin A), Vitamin E, and lecithin (plus other phosphatides), all required for the efficient digestion of fats and oils.

The experts say that linseed oil also metabolizes to prostaglandins. Prostaglandins play an important part in the heart function, regulate blood pressure, and assist in arterial functioning. In addition, linseed oil steps up the metabolic rate and assists in the vital oxygenation of every cell in the body. Proponents point out that it's this factor which is responsible for the steady increase of energy and the feelings of exhilaration and 'lightness' that regular users of linseed oil (with high-quality protein) experience.

THE ESSENTIAL FATS + PROTEIN

THE MAGIC COMBINATION — It really shouldn't take hundreds of years of scientific research to determine the optimum diet. All we really have to do is get back to the basics and eat the basic natural foods our bodies were designed to process as fuel. We have already discovered that linseeds contain the essential fatty acids, *plus* high-quality protein, *plus* the elements the body requires to process the essential fatty acids. Mother Nature does it right.

TRACKING THE EVIDENCE — Today's medical researchers owe a great deal to a number of early German biochemists and scientists. The discoveries these men made, outlined below, served as a shining beacon showing the way to today's scientific truths. In 1842, the brilliant chemistry professor Baron Justus von Liebig published work showing the relationship between the essential fatty acids and protein. In rapid succession came the studies of Eduard Pflueger (physiologist) in 1875, Ernst F. Hoppe-Seyler (physician and founder of the first published biochemical journal) in 1876, and the noted biochemist Lebedow in 1888. Working with laboratory animals, Lebedow proved that severely malnourished and starving animals died more quickly on a diet high in protein (without fats) or high in fats (without protein) than when given no food at all. But when the animals were given quality fats and protein together, they quickly recovered. The high quality fat that Lebedow selected was linseed oil.

In 1899, the brilliant scientist Rosenfeld took up the cause. Rosenfeld's experiments proved conclusively that consuming only animal fats led inescapably to fatty degeneration of the inner organs and obesity. Because the research identifying the difference between saturated animal fats and the essential fatty acids was many years in the future, Rosenfeld didn't know *why* this was so, but he proved conclusively that it *was* so. As Rosenfeld continued with his work on nutrition, he discovered

119

in 1902 that consuming a diet high in carbohydrates and low in protein resulted in fat deposits, as does a high carbohydrate, high protein diet. However, when he added high quality fats to the menu, his subjects slimmed down, lost their fat deposits, and had increased energy into the bargain. Rosenfeld had confirmed Lebedow's theory of 'good' fats (linseed oil) versus 'bad' fats (animal fats).

In 1920, Otto Meyerhof (1922 winner of the Nobel Prize for Physiology & Medicine) discovered that linoleic acid and sulphur-rich proteins form a natural partnership in the body. It was his work on cellular oxygenation and the transformation of lactic acid in muscles, created by the combination of essential fats and quality protein, that won him international recognition, the Nobel Prize, and assured his place in the annals of medicine. Albert Szent-Gyorgyi, a naturalized American of Hungarian descent (standing alone in the midst of the advanced German scientists), took the Nobel in 1937 for his further research on biological oxidation and ascorbic acid (Vitamin C). His work confirmed that linoleic acid, when combined with sulphur-based proteins, stimulates the oxygenation processes of the body. The 1931 Nobel Prize in Physiology & Medicine went to Otto Heinrich Warburg for his research proving that quality fats were required to repair the oxygenation function when it was depressed by fatty degeneration resulting in cancer and/or diabetes.

It was not until the late 20s and early 30s that the essential fatty acids, as we know them today, were isolated and identified by the noted scientists G. O. Burr and M. M. Burr. The results of their important work were published in 1929 in the *Journal of Biological Chemistry* (Volume 82: 345-367) and updated in the *Journal of Biological Chemistry* in 1930 (Volume 86: 587-621). Here's what they discovered. Working with laboratory animals, these two biochemists proved that animals fed a high protein diet which is severely deficient in the essential fatty acids die quickly. If the condition is not too advanced, they also showed that recovery was swift when the essential fats were put back into the diet.

This very promising line of research was neglected as the age of specialization dawned. Instead of continuing on with combinations of nutrients as their predecessors had done, the scientists of 50 years ago (and for most of the intervening years) narrowed their field of endeavor and concentrated on one nutrient at a time. Amino acids received the bulk of their attention.

In the mid 1950s, another brilliant German scientist took up where all the others had left off. Dr. Johanna Budwig (you'll learn all about her astounding breakthroughs in the treatment of cancer and the other diseases of fatty degeneration in the following chapter) has been battling commercial interests for thirty years. Using a combination of linseed oil and sulphur-based proteins, Dr. Budwig has proven conclusively that a return to the natural ways of eating can cure cancer. Do you think that this information was eagerly accepted by a waiting world desperately searching for a cancer cure? Not on your life! Recognizing the dangers of commercially manufactured dietary fats (margarine, hard shortening, vegetable oils), Dr. Budwig sought to publicize her findings, but found her way blocked by German manufacturers with a heavy financial stake in these products.

Dr. Budwig retired from public life and opened her own practice. She depends entirely on nutritional correction for her documented successes in curing cancer cases given up as terminal by the oxthodox medical community. You will read all about her findings in the following pages.

Chapter VI
The Miracle of Linseed Oil
The Medicinal Fat

A very good friend, George Friedrich, suffered three serious heart attacks between the ages of sixty and sixty-three. At the rate of one heart attack every year, his doctors didn't hold out much hope for a complete recovery. George's entire cardiovascular system was clogged with atherosclerotic plaque, interrupting the vital blood flow to his heart. He was put on very strong medication, including nitroglycerin for his angina pain, and was taking up to fifteen pills every day.

During the three years of his early sixties, George became very weak and aged visibly. He was on a downhill course until he was introduced to *Dr. Johanna Budwig's Formula*. He immediately incorporated Dr. Budwig's Formula into his daily diet. For breakfast every morning, he took 1 tablespoon of cold-processed, unrefined linseed oil mixed with low-fat cottage cheese. In order to make this fare more palatable, he added different herbs, raw vegetables, or fruits for variety. George found his favorite additions were a mixture of finely grated cucumbers and radishes with some chopped tomatoes.

After eating this low-fat cottage cheese 'salad' daily for just three months, George found his breathing was easing and the angina pain that had been with him for so long was almost eliminated. A year later, the medical doctors who examined him were amazed at his full recovery. Even his tiniest capillaries were as clean as those of a much younger man. Today, at age sixty-five, George no longer needs any pills. Needless to say, he is very grateful to have discovered Dr. Budwig's Formula in time.

LINSEED — PAST & PRESENT

THEN — Just what is this medicinal fat that forms the basis of Dr. Johanna Budwig's exclusive formula? You might be more familiar with linseed (Linum usitatissimum) as *flax*. Since prehistoric times, this graceful plant with its long, flat, elliptical seeds has been prized for its fibre, from which linen is made, and for the rich oil given up by its seeds.

Ayurvedic herbalists recognized the importance of linseed as a medicinal centuries ago. (*Ayurveda* is a very old Hindu system of natural medicine still practiced in some parts of Asia.) Herbologists consider the ripe oil-rich seeds of this botanical a superior internal demulcent (softening agent) and also use them in poultices for the treatment of rheumatism, gout, boils, and carbuncles. The oil is used as an enema to treat impacted feces. Mixed with lime water, the oil can be applied topically to promote the healing of skin lesions and to soothe the intolerable itch of eczema. The bark and leaves are believed to fight venereal diseases, especially gonorrhea.

The ancient Greeks and Romans used the brown, shiny seeds as a natural protein staple in their diet, and their ancestors followed suit as they spread across the entire European continent. The plant grows well in any temperate climate and was known in old India and parts of Russia, as well as South America and the early American colonies.

NOW — Linseed oil continues to be cultivated and is regarded as a high-quality vegetable oil in many parts of the world today, but most Americans look on it as merely an additive in oil-based paints or as livestock feed. In this country, the meal which remains after the oil is removed is compressed into cakes and used as a high-protein mineral-rich livestock food.

The central Europeans, in particular, value the healthful properties of this remarkable plant. Our cousins across the ocean can purchase *cold-pressed, virgin, unrefined raw linseed oil* as easily as we can purchase the over-processed, chemicalized and hydrogenated abominations that pass for vegetable oils lining the shelves of our local supermarkets.

THE OIL — Because the linseeds themselves contain from 33 to 43 percent oil, they give up their valuable liquid fat quite easily when compressed. When it hasn't been heated, filtered, and refined, the raw cold-processed linseed oil is a rich golden-yellow, amber, or brownish liquid. It thickens and becomes more viscous on exposure to air.

The light-colored refined variety which flows almost as easily as water, the only type of linseed oil available to the consumer currently in the U.S. (even in health food stores), has had all the valuable solid fats (the essential fatty acids the body requires) removed. Unfortunately, it cannot be considered an adequate substitute for the linseed oil we are discussing in this chapter.

RAW LINSEED OIL — In its *unrefined* form, linseed oil contains two important unsaturated fatty acids (linoleic and linolenic). When correctly processed, the oil consists of a healthy 58 percent essential fatty acids. These essential highly unsaturated fatty acids are converted in the body to *prostaglandins.*

In Europe, raw linseed oil is used therapeutically in the prevention and treatment of:

- **Cancer**
- **Arteriosclerosis** (reduces arteriosclerotic plaque/ cholesterol & triglyceride levels)
- **Strokes**
- **Cardiac Infarction**
- **Heartbeat** (irregular)
- **Red Blood Corpuscles** (maintains flexibility)
- **Liver** (fatty degeneration)
- **Lungs** (reduces bronchial spasms)

- **Intestines** (regulates activity)
- **Stomach Ulcers** (normalizes gastric juices)
- **Prostate** (hypertrophic)
- **Arthritis** (exerts a favorable influence)
- **Eczema** (assists all skin diseases)
- **Old Age** (improves many common afflictions)
- **Brain** (strengthens activity)
- **Immune Deficiency Syndromes** (cancer, multiple sclerosis, auto-immune illnesses)

Without essential fatty acids, prostaglandin biosynthesis cannot take place. The biological importance of prostaglandins lies in their high effectiveness, the range and diversity of their metabolic actions, and their wide distribution in the body. These chemically active substances affect the cardiovascular system, are present in the prostate gland, menstrual fluid, the brain, the lungs, the kidneys, the thymus gland, seminal fluid, and the pancreas. There are more than a dozen extremely important prostaglandins. All are derived from essential fatty acids. Without the essential fatty acids (present and active in raw linseed oil), the body cannot manufacture the prostaglandins it needs for healthy functioning. Considering the important part essential fatty acids play in manufacturing prostaglandins, it's easy to see why raw linseed oil is so therapeutically important.

WHO IS DR. JOHANNA BUDWIG?

As you learned in the previous chapter, it was Dr. Budwig who discovered that the right combination of essential fatty acids (potent and active in linseed oil) and sulphur-based proteins (present in abundance in low-fat cottage cheese) is the magic formula for conquering cancer and the other diseases of fatty degeneration. Dr. Johanna Budwig is known and highly respected around the world as Germany's premiere biochemist. In addition, Dr. Budwig holds a Ph.D. in Natural Science, has had medical training, and was schooled in pharmaceutical science, physics, botany and biology. In all courses, this brilliant scientist excelled. Here's how Dr. Budwig's momentous discovery came about:

Building on the early findings of her colleagues (as outlined in the previous chapter), three decades ago, Dr. Budwig began systematic research into the problems of fatty degeneration. The refinements in investigative medical techniques she needed for the type of analysis she envisioned were not available, so she developed them. Thanks to Dr. Budwig's pioneering efforts, the elements present in a single drop of blood can now be isolated and identified. She was on her way to solving the mysteries of fat metabolism and close to an incredible breakthrough in medical science.

Dr. Budwig began collecting and meticulously analyzing literally thousands of blood samples, both from healthy specimens and from the seriously ill. The data that she tabulated showed that blood of the seriously ill (including cancer patients, diabetics, those with precancerous conditions of the liver) was always, without exception, deficient in one of the important essential fatty acids (linoleic acid). Other deficiencies became apparent as well. Also missing were phosphatides (required for normal cell division), and albumin (a blood producing lipoprotein).

Without the normalizing phosphatides, cancer cells (an abnormality) grow wild and proliferate. Without albumin (a combination of linoleic acid and sulphur-based protein), blood analysis shows a strange chartreuse (greenish-yellow) substance in place of the healthy red oxygen-carrying hemoglobin that belongs there. This fact explains why cancer patients are weakened and anemic. Without linoleic acid, the body can't produce hemoglobin. Without hemoglobin, the blood is unable to carry vital oxygen to the suffocating cells and tissues. Energy production suffers; the cancer victim becomes progressively more and more anemic, sinks into lethargy, and finally dies.

The blood of a healthy person always contains sufficient quality protein and the essential fatty acids. Progressing from this point of fact, Dr. Budwig reasoned that the victims of the diseases of fatty degeneration could be restored to health by supplying a diet high in essential fatty acids and sulphur-based proteins.

To test her theory, Dr. Budwig determined to begin with the highest-quality oil available in all nature. With its rich content of linoleic and linolenic acids (both the essential fatty acids), the liquid gold of crude linseed oil fit that description perfectly. For the sulphur-based proteins, Dr. Budwig selected skim milk. (Note: The latest Budwig formula uses low-fat cottage cheese in place of skim milk). She fed seriously ill cancer patients a combination of 100 grams of skim milk proteins with 40 grams of fresh linseed oil. To make the mixture easier to blend (and swallow), she added 25 grams of milk. During the period of these early experiments, she drew blood and analyzed the samples constantly, looking closely for the most minute changes.

What she found was gratifying indeed. Over a period of approximately three months, tumors gradually receded. The strange greenish elements in the blood were replaced with healthy red blood cells as the phosphatides and lipoproteins almost miraculously reappeared. The anemia disappeared and life-energy was restored. Symptoms of cancer, liver dysfunction, and diabetes were completely alleviated. Today, after ten years of solid clinical application, Dr. Budwig's cottage cheese and linseed oil formula has been proven successful where many orthodox remedies have failed.

Because of the influence of the powerful oil processing industry in Germany (which continues to attempt to discredit her findings), she was denied publication in medical journals. Dr. Budwig has published her research on the properties and benefits of linseed oil under various titles, including *"Cancer — A Fat Problem," "The Death of the Tumour,"* and *"True Health Against Arteriosclerosis, Heart Infarction, & Cancer."* (Note: These books are available as German language editions only and are not published in English.) Dr. Budwig has assisted many seriously ill individuals, even those given up as terminal by orthodox medical practitioners, to regain their health through a simple regimen of nutrition. The basis of Dr. Budwig's program is the use of linseed oil blended with cottage cheese.

Because her research has been highly publicized in Europe, even the man on the street has long been aware of the dangers of consuming too much of the wrong kind of fat. To illustrate this point, Dr. Budwig tells a charming story published in the *London Daily Express* headlined "Fat In Your Frying Pan Can Kill."

A husband returning home from an exhausting day at work said to his wife, "Pan fry me a steak, dear, but throw the fat away." "Certainly, not!" replied his wife. "The fat I'll use to crisp your steak the way you like it cost 36 cents! Do you really want me to throw away 36 cents?" The husband, in mock horror, answered, "What! Your husband isn't worth 36 cents to you?"

Dr. Budwig teaches that the way in which the body metabolizes fat concerns every vital organ in the body, pointing out that people afflicted with liver and gallbladder problems in particular cannot tolerate fat. She also observes that a high-fat diet doesn't agree with any unhealthy person, but explains that the three-times unsaturated, oxygenated fats in linseed oil, when taken with protein-rich cottage cheese, are easily tolerated by anyone, even those seriously ill.

Dr. Budwig tells of giving a lecture in Switzerland to hundreds of people. As she was taking questions from the audience, a man and wife approached the podium and asked to tell the listeners of their experiences. Dr. Budwig passed the man the microphone. He told of his daughter who had a serious deterioration of one knee joint. Her doctors had said her condition was incurable, that medical science had no hope for her, that she would eventually be completely bedridden and, unable to care for herself, would require full-time nursing care in a sanitorium. The unfortunate young girl also suffered from a disfiguring case of psoriasis. The man said that he himself had a tumor in one lung and went on to tell of the health problems of his son. He then passed the microphone to his wife and she completed the story. She said that when she began insisting the entire family follow Dr. Budwig's recommendation to eat linseed oil with cottage cheese every day, gradually their health improved. She reported that all four members of the family regained complete and robust health on Dr. Budwig's simple regimen.

DR. JOHANNA BUDWIG SPEAKS

Dr. Budwig lectures all over Europe. Her fame precedes her and she is acclaimed on the continent for her important work. Thousands flock to hear her speak whenever she appears. The many people she has helped revere her and testify to the benefits of her simple program of health. During my recent trip to Europe in early 1986, I had the privilege of interviewing Dr. Budwig and learned first-hand of her exciting approach to the cure and treatment of cancer, heart infarction, arteriosclerosis, stroke, and other problems of fatty degeneration. I have spoken with Dr. Budwig at length, have studied her published research material, and read her many books with keen interest. We have had a wealth of her printed material translated into the English language and excerpt as follows:

"As far back as 1957, the Cancer Research Institute of Paris, France began studies to determine the exact differences between a cancer cell and a normal cell. As revealed during the International Congress of Nutrition, the French scientists announced that they had found a lot of undissolved fat deposited in the nucleus, body, and plasma of the cancer cell. In his book, *The Cancer Problem,* Professor Bauer of Germany said that fat can both dissolve tumors and cause tumors. Although at the time this statement appeared contradictory, we know now that there are many different types of fat.

"Following this line of reasoning, it is obvious that if we feed the body the highly unsaturated and oxygenated essential fatty acids it requires, along with the high quality protein which makes fat easily soluble, it will counteract toxic and poisonous accumulations in the tissues. If we also stay away from chemical preservatives, then many, many people will become healthy very fast — even some who have been given up by doctors and hospitalized to die. I have proved this premise many times.

129

"Every part of the body is affected adversely by the use of saturated fats, including the brain, the liver, the kidneys, and the nervous system. But the function of the heart is perhaps the hardest hit when a disturbance in the fat metabolism occurs. When the wrong kind of fat has been ingested, it is transported via the blood and lymph. Fat globules (atherosclerotic plaque) are deposited in these vital pathways leading to heart disease.

"Poor nutrition gives rise to many problems. For instance, I once visited a woman in Switzerland who was suffering from terminal cancer. As a mother, her main concern was not herself, but the health of her two children, a boy of 12 and girl of 14. Both were obese and looked ill. I gathered the little family together and spoke to them of the importance of eating correctly. The daughter said to me in a soft voice, 'What is this wonderful preparation that can make us all well?' I explained how to prepare a cottage cheese salad dressed with linseed oil and how it could benefit the entire household.

"On the whole, I blame the older generation for the generally poor health of so many. Foods are commonly overprocessed and chemical additives are used to extend the shelf life and make more money for the manufacturers. The wrong kinds of fats are used and they are not pure. Many sexual dysfunctions are caused because the body cannot metabolize these foods. Fortunately, many health problems can be easily remedied simply by correcting the diet.

"When I talk about my linseed oil/high-quality protein fare, it is nothing but a simple food which contains the most active fat known to me: linseed oil. In this form, the essential fatty acids are easily assimilated and made soluble in connection with essential amino acids (protein) in the form of cottage cheese. This is good-tasting and very palatable. It has been used in Europe for many years by hundreds of thousands of individuals.

"I tell you now that this simple food can inhibit the growth of tumors. By completely natural means, fat metabolism is stimulated and the size of the tumor actually decreases. Of course, it is better that you not wait until three or four doctors and several hospitals have told you that your tumor is incurable. Instead, regain maximum health by always using the best nutrition. In a very short period of time, even the most seriously ill person will feel better.

"Very often I go into hospitals and take home very seriously sick cancer patients who have been told they don't have long to live. The first improvement which encourages these sick people and their families is when they say things like: 'In the hospital, I couldn't urinate.' 'In the hospital, I couldn't have a bowel movement.' 'In the hospital, I couldn't clear the mucus from my throat.' Suddenly all those blockages clear and the system becomes activated again simply because the linseed oil and cottage cheese I give are rich in essential fatty acids and electrons which emulsify the blockages and remove them. Sick people tell me, 'I feel so much lighter and not dragged down and heavy any more.'

"We have to return to this immune biological way of eating. I have been to Japan, China, and even India attending many scientifically oriented symposiums and have connections with many researchers in this field. They all wonder the same thing: 'Why is it that the biological approach of treating disease is so often attacked by authorities in the orthodox medical field?' I myself have been to court many times to defend my beliefs. Fortunately, all courts ruled in my favor.

"What is it that I am doing? It's very simple. If any cancer patient comes to me, I just give them simple, natural nutrition. That's all. What can we learn from all this?

"First, we must restore correct nutrition. Fats, proteins, fruits, and vegetables are very important. But we have to be careful to take them in an unrefined and totally natural state, as nature intended.

"Second, we should be careful to avoid foods which have been contaminated with chemicals through processing or refining or treatment with antibiotics and growth hormones.

"To stay healthy and maintain all the vital functions of the body we absolutely must be able to metabolize fat efficiently. The continuing research on fat metabolism in connection with oxygenation, absorption, and assimilation of energy is of immense importance. If we are to survive in the western civilized world as a human being and a race, it's time to think about living our lives through sound biological principles.

"The secret of the wisdom of the universe is that science must conform with nature. Science and nature must work in harmony. Time is running out for all of us. We must begin to think and act and, most importantly, eat responsibly for the health and welfare of the race."

FATS AFFECT EVERY PART OF THE BODY

Dr. Budwig appears to have discovered one of the most important secrets of regaining or maintaining health. Consider: When we compare a healthy heart with one that has just suffered a heart attack, we find that the diseased heart is burdened with an accumulation of fat. A victim of arthritis carries excessive fatty deposits in his aching joints and muscles, but a healthy person does not. An organ attacked by cancer commonly shows an infiltration of yellowish-white fat globules with the appearance of tiny cauliflower-like rosettes.

The first visible symptom of cancer is the separation of lipids (fats) from the surrounding tissue. Saturated, hydrogenated, chemically hardened fats can actually act as chemical carcinogens within the body. Dr. Budwig's research indicates that the trouble begins when the protein-bound fats, normally present as free-flowing lipids in a live organism, become separated from their protein carriers and end up as unhealthy deposits in various parts of the body.

FATS ARE IMPORTANT — Science has proven that fats play an important part in the functioning of the entire body. Fats (lipids) are vital for all growth processes, renewal of cells, brain and nerve functions, even for the sensory organs (eyes and ears), and for the body's adjustment to heat, cold, and quick temperature changes. Our energy resources are based on lipid metabolism.

Each and every cell in this miracle we call the body is protectively covered with a sheath of fats. The cell body (plasma) is interlaced with little lipid veins, often called the 'nerves of the cell.' These lipid nerve-veins are the connection between the nucleus and the outer membrane. They influence the care and feeding of the cell and the process of normal cell division by the use of tiny electrical impulses. To function efficiently, cells require polyunsaturated live *electron-rich* lipids, present in abundance in crude linseed oil. Polyunsaturated fats greedily absorb proteins and oxygen. It is a documented fact that many people suffer from an oxygen shortage simply because they are deficient in these oxygen-active lipids.

Lipids are only water-soluble and free-flowing when bound to protein, thus forming an electric counterpole to their protein carriers. This vitally important type of fat contains accumulated energy in its electron clouds. When high quality electron-rich fats are combined with proteins, the electrons are protected until the body requires energy. This energy source is fully and immediately available to the body on demand, as nature intended. These energy resources can be instantly mobilized and rushed into action as needed.

The presence of these important lipids can be compared to the capital (money reserves) of a corporation. Any type of growth or activity, whether that of a corporation or the human body, requires an expenditure of capital (money or energy). In the body, any activity (physical or mental) or growth factor (during pregnancy or the normal growing period from infant to adult, for example) requires the presence of electron-rich fats bound to proteins. All the cells, muscle masses, brain, nerves, organs, and lifestreams (blood and lymph) of the body need these electrically-charged, highly-active lipids. The demands on these energy reserves are enormous. Every breath we take, every muscle we move, every time the heart beats — even the automatic process of renewal and division of every cell in the body — depends on this energy source.

Let's examine the benefits accruing to the heart from electrically-charged lipids. There is an immediate harmonious interaction with the heart when the spent venous blood receives a healthy dose of lipids from the lymphatic system immediately before entering the heart. Inside the heart, the venous blood and lipids are mixed, creating a measurable electric current which regulates the action of the heart and sends impulses to the entire circulatory system. This blood, now charged by the electron-rich lipids, then flows to the lungs where it is charged with oxygen and pumped through the left ventricle into the aortas of the body. The vital life-sustaining pumping action of the heart itself depends on the electrical charge created by the lipids.

Some highly respected oncologists (cancer specialists) have pointed out that the bio-oxidation of the cell is seriously inhibited in a malignant tumor. As bio-oxidation decreases, fermentation metabolism of the cancerous cell increases. The antioxidants used in the chemically processed oils and margarines we put on the family table obstruct the bio-oxidation of every cell in the body. However, virgin linseed oil *(cold-processed, unrefined, and additive-free)* actually stimulates the bio-oxidation of cells and tissues and normalizes the important oxygenation processes throughout the organism.

The frequent successes which have been obtained in treatment with the essential fatty acids and the lipotropic effect' of essential amino acids brings us quickly to the realization that only a combination of essential proteins with essential fatty acids can bring about the full beneficial impact of these vital elements.

THE IMPORTANT FOODS — Many of the foods we commonly eat are lacking in both essential fatty acids and essential amino acids. The essential amino acids (proteins) are present in abundance in cottage cheese, buttermilk, hard cheeses, whole wheat, fish, and lean meats. The essential fatty acids the body hungers for are found in rich supply in crude, unrefined linseed oil, soy lecithin, egg yolks, and some vegetable oils. The problem, of course, with most commercially processed vegetable oils that stock the shelves of our supermarkets is that they are heated, refined, hydrogenated, and full of chemical preservatives. Because the essential fatty acids are particularly sensitive to heat and oxidation, margarines and processed vegetable oils no longer carry their content of essential fatty acids. (See Chapter 5.)

It is only when the body is well supplied with the essential fatty acids and essential amino acids in proper balance that the metabolic system can function as nature intends that it should. In the presence of these vital elements, healthy oxygenated blood courses richly throughout the entire organism to benefit every cell. When the essential fatty acids bind with the essential amino acids, the offspring of this happy marriage are called 'lipoproteids.' Healthy people have an abundance of lipoproteids, but it has been observed that diseased patients (including victims of cancer) have a much reduced level of lipoproteids in their blood, or none at all.

By comparing the body to a wood or coal burning stove, perhaps we can form an easily understood mental picture, albeit very simplified, of the workings of the body. Let's say that the stove has been overheated often, it has been fed the cheapest grade of coal, and its maintenance has been neglected for a long period of time. The body of the stove, the stovepipe, and the chimney become clogged with a dangerous residue that could flare into flames at any time, and which might very well burn down the house. We must clean away the deposits and feed the stove well-dried wood that burns cleanly without leaving a harmful residue.

The body which has been wrongly fed, poorly maintained, and neglected is in the same sad state as the abused stove. Harmful deposits and a residue of fats clog the inner workings of the body. By introducing the clean essential fatty acids present in linseed oil and the superior high quality proteins (amino acids) present in cottage cheese, the body immediately goes to work to rid itself of the deposits inhibiting its normal functioning. By continuing to feed the body with these good natural nutrients, soon the body becomes healthy again as nature intended.

Needless to say, after the body (or the stove) has been efficiently cleansed and is free of harmful deposits, we're certainly not going to return to the same old suspect foods that caused the problem in the first place. In order to stay well, the experts say that good dietary habits must be followed rigorously for a lifetime.

EXAMINING CHEMICALLY PROCESSED FATS — Dr. Johanna Budwig preaches against the use of what she calls

135

'pseudo' fats. In order to extend the shelf life, to provide the market with a visually attractive assortment of liquid and artificially hardened fats (margarines) — in short, to make money manufacturers use chemical processes that render their products harmful to the body. These fats may be marked 'polyunsaturated,' but they are damaging to the body all the same. If you doubt the truth of this statement, please go back and review Chapter 5 carefully.

The chemical processing of fats destroys the vital electron cloud, demonstrated in the foregoing material to be of immense importance to the functioning of every cell in the body. Once the electrons have been removed, these fats can no longer bind with oxygen and actually become an obstacle to the process of breathing. The heart, for instance, rejects these fats and they end up as inorganic fatty deposits on the heart muscle itself. As we pointed out earlier, a diseased heart and its aortas clearly show deposits of these worthless, electrically dead lipids.

Chemically processed fats are not water-soluble when bound to protein. They end up blocking circulation, damage heart action, inhibit cell renewal, and impede the free flow of blood and lymph fluids. The bio-electrical action in these areas slows down and may become completely paralyzed. The entire organism shows a measurable loss of the electrical energy which is replenished only by adding active lipids to the diet. These nutritional fats are truly vital for man and beast alike.

In recent years, scientists have coined the term 'fat intolerance' and deplore the damage done by fat degeneration. It's hard to believe that science hasn't discovered the root of the problem. The body rejects chemically processed fats because their composition has been changed so drastically from what nature intended that they are no longer able to fulfill their function in the organism, but instead cause untold damage to the body.

It is interesting to note that Russia outlawed the chemical saturation of fats for the purpose of causing them to harden artificially, as in the production of margarine, as long ago as 1902. Dr. Budwig explains that it is impossible to correct the damage done to lipids once they have been hardened into margarine just by adding some linoleic acid. In order to obtain a high level of linoleic acid, the manufacturers put in a chemical combination of ethyl and methyl esters, not the pure natural oil. Much research has documented the fact that this type of artificial linoleic acid does not combat the symptoms of an essential fatty acid deficiency in the body.

In direct contrast to the chemically produced fatty acids, consider what happens when just a minute quantity (one microgram) of linseed oil is introduced into the bloodstream of a cancer patient. Because the natural fatty acids present in crude linseed oil easily bind with oxygen and protein, the blood of the cancer patient improves within four to six hours. The activity of these natural lipids in the blood stream can actually be microscopically observed.

Fat damage is apparent in the heart, the liver, the arteries, and is clearly visible in malignant (and benign) tumors. The source of this degenerative damage lies in faulty nutrition, in the intake of the wrong kinds of fats. These findings have been substantiated by cancer researchers from twenty-nine NATO countries. Surely, no health-care practitioner, no scientist, and no thinking person can continue to ignore the facts. The essential electronically-charged fats that are found in abundance in natural linseed oil are crucially important to the health and functioning of the body.

Dr. Budwig herself teaches that the most favorable way to attack cancer at its roots is by removing all 'pseudo' fats from the diet and introducing the true nutrition of the natural medicinal fats present in linseed oil.

HIGH FAT CONSUMPTION — Are the citizens of the civilized world consuming too much of the wrong kind of fat? Statistics show that overall fat consumption is on the rise. Research conducted with laboratory animals has given us an important insight into one of the metabolic disorders arising from the overconsumption of saturated fats. Lab animals fed a diet high in saturated fats greedily consume as much as five to six times as much food (including fats) as animals fed a normal diet. Even more important, this study showed that when the animals were fed natural fats from linseeds, they consumed only about one-fifth of the fat and one-fifth of other foods in comparison with the group of animals fed saturated fats.

This experiment showed very graphically that 'cheap' fats are actually very expensive, both in terms of cost and in terms of health. In an effort to ingest the essential fatty acids their bodies craved, the lab animals ate five times as much of the commercially processed fats as did the animals supplied with the electron-rich active natural fats. This may very well be the explanation of just *why* our overall fat consumption is increasing. After all, the human body is not so very different from the body of an animal bred for laboratory research.

The health and well-being of the organism depends entirely on the type of nutrition consumed. Research has demonstrated that normal growth, healthy skin, glandular functions (liver, gall bladder, pancreas, stomach, intestines, prostate, lymph), are especially dependent on active fats. Glandular secretions are dependent on natural protein-reactive lipids. When chemically processed fats (protein and oxygen inactive) are consumed, there is a consequent inhibiting of all glandular activity within the system.

One of the first symptoms of faulty fat metabolism, easily observed by any of us, is a drying of the mucuous membranes of the nose and mouth. The dried-out mucuous membranes of the typical cancer patient, resulting in a sore, raspy voice, are caused when the glandular secretions are inhibited by the ingestion of chemically processed fats. Not so easily recognized, but just as harmful, is the drying effect exerted on the entire digestive and intestinal tract.

QUICK IMPROVEMENT — After only two weeks on the Johanna Budwig regimen of high quality protein and electron-rich linseed oil with its essential fats, the emaciated patient starts to gain weight consistently as his appetite returns. From being resigned to an early death, his feelings change to the joyous anticipation of recovery. An improvement in glandular and mucous secretions in all upper and lower body cavities, including improved intestinal functioning, can be observed in mere days, sometimes in just a few hours. Both asthma sufferers and those with cancer of the tongue have found quick and profound help.

Critical observers have tried to label this phenomenon as a psychotherapeutic (mind-induced) effect. However, Dr. Budwig points to her years of observation of psychologically impartial patients. These patients have testified to the truth of their own well-being and state their cures were accomplished by a simple change in diet. Dr. Budwig's patients want to talk about the so-called 'incurable' tumor which disappeared, the weakened and debilitated muscles which became firm, the seriously affected digestive system which was normalized after only a few days on her regimen, the painful and irregular menstrual periods which became normal, the most advanced case of cancer of the colon which healed. Dr. Budwig says that, as the internal functions of the body are normalized, even the smell of the patient's stool becomes less foul. Swelling and edema disappear as normal urination patterns are again established. The cancer patient begins to live again as he experiences the return of well-being. Very soon, he is free of pain without the use of strong medication or injections.

WORLD-WIDE RESEARCH

THE USE OF LINSEED OIL — Linseed oil is an edible poly-unsaturated vegetable oil and is used in cooking in many parts of the world. It is very rich in essential polyunsaturated fats (linoleic and linolenic acids). Because these fatty acids are known to be essential to the body, many researchers around the world are investigating their properties and trying to determine the benefits of adding linseed oil to the diet. The current research coming out of Europe can benefit us all by pointing the way to both a preventive and therapeutic approach to many diseases. The results reported by various scientific authorities, excerpted below, are truly astounding.

GREAT BRITAIN — This very interesting study entitled *Changes in the Rumen Metabolism of Sheep Given Increasing Arounts of Linseed Oil in Their Diet* gives an indication of the function of linseed oil and how it can benefit the body.

We quote, "It appears that the lowering of the concentration of acetate in the rumen was not the result of decreased production, but rather increased utilization, such as one would expect if lipid synthesis increased. Linseed oil added to the diet did not depress VFA (volatile fatty acid) production, but actually increased it. Results confirmed that up to 25 grams of additional lipids could be synthesized by supplying linseed oil with the sheeps' diet."

A 'translation' follows. *Acetate* is a substance produced in the body when fats are not properly metabolized. However, when linseed oil was added to their diet, the contents of the sheeps' *rumen* (first stomach) showed that, even on this extremely high-fat feed, the *lipids* (fats) were being efficiently used.

POLAND — In a paper entitled *The Cytotoxic Action of Unsaturated Fatty acids on Cancer,* the Department of Pharmaceutical Technology of the Medical Academy, Wroclaw, Poland, announced: "The fatty acids isolated from linseed oil were found to exhibit a strong cytotoxic in vitro activity against Ehrlich ascites cancer cells with minimal cytotoxic effect on normal cells (leukocytes) of the peritoneal exudate in rabbits. The fatty acids from linseed oil (1000 g/ml after a 3 hour incubation) gave 100 percent dead carcinoma cells."

In plain English, the near-miraculous news is that the active elements of linseed oil exerted a *cytotoxic* (cell destroying) action against cancer cells *in vitro* (literally, in 'glass,' as in a test tube or lab dish), but bypassed healthy *leukocytes* (white blood cells).

POLAND — In yet another study, scientists working at the Institute of Pharmacology & Toxicology at the Medical Academy confirm that linoleic acid has anti-thrombotic (anti-clotting) effects in animals and man. This report concluded that, "Replacement of dietary saturated fatty acids by linoleic acid lowers the risk for myocardial infarction as well as cardiovascular death rate. The cholesterol lowering effect of linoleic acid was clearly demonstrated."

GERMANY — From the Department of Pharmacology & Toxicology, Martin Luther University in Wittenberg, Germany, comes a research paper entitled *The Influence of a Linseed Oil Diet on Fatty Acid Patterns in Phospholipids & Thromboxane Formation in Platelets in Man.*

Interest in mounting this study developed due to the fact that Greenland Eskimos, who traditionally eat a diet high in EPA (known to increase the metabolism of fat), rarely suffer from heart disease. Building on the work of G. Hornstra (as published in Lancet, 1979), the bottom line is that this paper demonstrates that a diet rich in linseed oil can lower the risk of arterial thrombosis.

Noting that "A linseed oil diet is known as a 'prudent diet' in Germany," the scientists reported: "A diet of linseed oil (30 ml daily) for four weeks raised the content of linolenic acid by twofold, of EPA (eicosapentaenoic acid) by 150 percent, and of docosahexaenoic acid by 70 percent in the serum of volunteers. The human body seems capable of transforming linolenic acid into EPA. This change coincided with a significantly reduced production of platelet thromboxanes (clotting agents)."

INDIA — The Department of Medicine, Patna Medical College & Hospital, Patna, India, has released the results of a study entitled *Influence of Linseed Oil on Cholesterol-Induced Atherosclerosis in Rabbits.* Beginning with the premise that many researchers have shown that saturated fats increase the severity of atherosclerosis, the Indian doctors adminstered 25 g linseed oil with their feed to 36 albino rabbits for a period of 18 weeks.

At the close of the experiment, the animals were sacrificed and the researchers reported: "Atherosclerotic lesions were absent in group L (fed linseed oil), but the percentage of atherosclerotic lesions was significantly high in the control groups (not given linseed oil)."

It is important to note that in the group of animals given PUFA (polyunsaturated fatty acids) along with a cholesterol-inducing diet of saturated fats, a greater incidence of cholesterol buildup was noted. Of this statistic, the scientists say: "The hypercholesterolemic effect of (the combination of) saturated *and* unsaturated fat in rabbits fed cholesterol is caused by increased absorption and retention of cholesterol."

Does this mean that all polyunsaturated fats are not created equal? Apparently so. Linseed oil itself is a highly polyunsaturated fat, but did not contribute to a buildup of harmful cholesterol or atherosclerotic plaque.

AUSTRALIA — Coming to us from the Royal Perth Hospital of the University of Western Australia 'down under,' is a study entitled *An Inhibitory Effect of Dietary Polyunsaturated Fatty Acids (PUFAs) on Renin Secretion in the Isolated Perfused Rat Kidney.* In case you're confused, slowing down (inhibiting) the production of *renin,* is good. Renin is a protein that masquerades as an enzyme and acts as a powerful *vasoconstrictor* (compressing the veins and restricting the vital free flow of blood).

Excerpting from this paper: "After a four-week regimen of diets enriched with linseed oil, safflower oil, or saturated fat (providing 20 percent of the total daily energy intake), the animals fed linseed oil showed a significant fall in the proportion of arachidonic acid in renal phospholipids (kidney fats) and a reduction in urinary prostaglandin excretion. In comparison with the other dietary groups, linseed oil feeding also resulted in a consistently lower renal vascular tone. Results suggest that dietary enrichment with PUFAs may contribute to the lower blood pressures observed." In theory, it might be said that the superior effects of the linseed oil diet are related to increased vasodilator (vein expansion) activity.

Another study from the same source entitled *Dietary Modification of Platelet & Renal Prostaglandins* provides a clearer explanation of the lowered blood pressure readings observed, as follows: "Changes in renal (kidney) function and blood pressure control were reversed by restoring essential fatty acids to the diet. Dietary linseed oil caused the incorporation of linolenic acid into plasma and kidney lipids with a relatively minor reduction in arachidonic acid when compared to the hydrogenated coconut oil control. Diets rich in linoleic acid have also been shown to delay the onset of hypertension (high blood pressure).

"Prostaglandins are synthesized from arachidonic acid which, in turn, is produced from dietary linoleic acid.

Prostaglandins are involved in a number of blood pressure regulating mechanisms and have potent direct vascular effects. Significant changes in fatty acid and prostaglandin metabolism can be achieved with fat supplements of less than 40 percent of energy. Rats on an oil-rich diet showed an average lower blood pressure than animals on the standard diet."

FRANCE — The National Institute of Alimentary Research, Dijon Cedex, France, has published a report entitled *The Transference of Cyclic Monomeric Acids into the Milk of Rats Ingesting Thermopolymerized Linseed Oil*. The results of this study of pregnant and nursing female rats fed linseed oil interjects a cautionary note into the otherwise unblemished record of dietary linseed oil.

The researchers found that the administration of linseed oil (100 g of linseed oil thermopolymerized at 275 degrees centigrade per kilogram of feed) to female rats during the period of gestation and lactation caused the death of all young, either at birth or in the two weeks following birth. Rats on a regular commercial diet up to the day of littering gave birth to normal young. When these same females were given linseed oil in their diet during the nursing period, the young rats did not die, but their rate of growth was measurably slowed.

WARNING: Although the amount of linseed oil fed the female rats in this study was proportionately much greater than would normally be ingested by a pregnant woman supplementing her diet with this nutrient, the results of this important research certainly indicate that *a women who is (or suspects she might be) pregnant should not include linseed oil in her diet until after giving birth and weaning the child.*

AUSTRALIA — The Microbiology Department of the Royal Melbourne Hospital in Victoria, Australia published a paper in 1981 entitled *Anti-bacterial Activity of Hydrolysed Linseed Oil & Linolenic Acid Against Methicillin-Resistant Staphylococcus Aureus (MSRA)*.

We quote: "Methicillin-resistant strains of Staphylococcus aureus, which are also resistant to most other anti-staphylococcal antibiotics, are currently causing a widespread epidemic of hospital-acquired infection in the State of Victoria. Patients who are colonized with MRSA appear to run a greater risk of infection after operative or other invasive procedures than do those who lack these strains.

"For many strains (of MRSA) at low concentrations of linolenic acid and hydrolysed linseed oil, there was a striking reduction in the size of the colonies. Our data show that MRSA are sensitive to hydrolysed linseed oil as well as linolenic acid. Preparations containing hydrolysed linseed oil may have a role in the eradication of the staphylococcal carrier state and could also be useful for prophylaxis, especially in debilitated patients."

Not only in Australia, but all over the world, the risk of contracting a staph infection while in a hospital is very real. This landmark report on the antibacterial effects of linseed oil (and linolenic acid) should be given world-wide attention.

AUSTRIA — The German publication *Research & Technology* (Forschung und Technik) recently reported on a three year study being conducted in Austria. Armed with a government grant, several Austrian biochemists and local teaching hospitals in the area have combined forces to investigate the properties of linseed oil against cancer.

Beginning with the basic research and fundamental data of Dr. Johanna Budwig, the Austrian scientists acclaimed Dr. Budwig's successful cures of cancer patients over the past ten years. Because linseed oil has been shown to inhibit the proliferation of malignant cells, these medical authorities are adding their voice to those who call this miracle oil "a glimmer of hope in the fight against cancer." This three-year study, already showing that the application of the highly unsaturated fats in linseed oil works against cancer, is proceeding as planned.

SOME HEARTWARMING STORIES

The foregoing reports of laboratory research scientifically document the benefits of linseed oil, but make very dry reading. On a personal level, the following stories are representative of the wonders that crude linseed oil combined with high quality protein can work in the lives of real people.

Coming out of Europe, and most especially stemming from the work of German biochemist Dr. Johanna Budwig, we hear astounding reports on the great benefits of simply adding linseed oil to the diet. Dr. Budwig reports that the essential fatty acids present in raw, cold-processed, unrefined linseed oil require a powerful supply of concentrated protein (amino acids) in order to efficiently metabolize in the body. Dr. Budwig's recommended regimen of using one tablespoon of raw, unrefined linseed oil drizzled over one-half cup of protein-rich cottage cheese (please select the low-fat variety) daily apparently works wonders. Read on.

MALIGNANT OSTEOMA — Magda W. tells her story in her own words: "I was told by the most expert doctors that I would have to be operated on to cut out the cancerous tumor that was causing a swelling under my eye. They explained that the size of the tumor was much greater inside and that there was very serious bone involvement. The malignancy was too far advanced to respond to radiation treatment. The doctors planned to remove considerable facial tissue and bone. I was afraid for my life, but being a young woman, couldn't bear the thought of such disfigurement.

"When I heard about Dr. Budwig's linseed oil and protein diet, I was skeptical but desperate for help. After four months on this regimen, the swelling under my left eye completely disappeared. The doctors at the University Hospital gave me many exhausting tests. One told me, 'If I didn't have your previous x-rays and medical history in front of me, I wouldn't believe that you had ever had cancer. There is hardly any indication of a tumor remaining.' I never thought that using Dr. Budwig's formula would be so successful. My whole family and I are very grateful."

BASAL CELL CARCINOMA — An elderly woman of 76 years of age, Mrs. Erika H., was afflicted with a somewhat slow-growing cancer on the tip of her nose which nevertheless was developing into a particularly ugly and disfiguring *rodent ulcer*. (A rodent ulcer is a gnawing cancer which eats through soft tissue and bone.) Because of Mrs. H.'s advanced age and the site of the cancer, her physician was understandably reluctant to operate and was attempting to treat her in the traditional manner.

Although Mrs. H. disliked being seen in public, a neighbor persuaded her to attend a lecture given by Dr. Johanna Budwig which was being held in a nearby town. After hearing Dr. Budwig speak, Mrs. H. began taking the linseed oil/cottage cheese combination religiously, adding a few cooking herbs from her kitchen garden to overcome the oily taste. She also applied linseed oil directly to the site of the cancer every evening before retiring. Very slowly, the affected tissue on the tip of her nose began to regenerate and eventually the ulcer healed. Mrs. H.'s physician credits modern medical techniques, but Mrs. H. herself believes with all her heart that Dr. Budwig's 'recipe for health' was responsible for her near-miraculous cure.

HODGKIN'S DISEASE — At the tender age of seven years, young Tommy G. was sent to the Children's Hospital where he was diagnosed as having Hodgkin's Disease. The child was operated on and underwent 24 radiation treatments, plus additional experimental therapies that the experts hoped would be of some small help. When Tommy failed to respond favorably to these heroic measures, he was discharged as incurable and sent home. His sorrowing parents were told his life expectancy was less than six months.

While in the hospital, Tommy had gone from a sturdy little boy into an emaciated and frail figure. His arms and legs were so thin that the outline of his bones were clearly visible. He had burns and scars on his neck, under both arms, and in his groin from the many radiation treatments he had undergone. His voice was hoarse and his breathing labored. After only a few weeks, this unfortunate youngster lost his ability to speak entirely. The ear, nose, and throat specialist the parents consulted told them that Tommy's vocal cords had been severely burned by the radiation treatments. He was admitted to the hospital again, this time to die.

The desperate parents contacted specialists all over the world, including Europe, Switzerland, and America. A famous newspaper took up Tommy's cause and ran editorials pleading for someone to come forth who could offer hope for the child's life. All the specialists who replied confirmed the cruel prognosis: There was no hope or help for Tommy. At this dark hour, the miracle the family had prayed for happened!

Tommy's mother told their story for the press: "A friend sent me a printed piece about one of Dr. Budwig's speeches. This material gave us hope and I contacted Dr. Budwig. I wanted to give my boy her diet in the hospital clinic, but the doctors told me they didn't have time for this special attention. We took Tommy home and started him on the diet ourselves. I kept in close touch with Dr. Budwig. In just five days, Tommy's breathing became normal for the first time in almost two years. Three weeks later, his voice came back. From this day on, Tommy began to feel good again. He went back to school, started swimming, and by winter, he was doing craft work. He will soon be twelve years old and is now a healthy, happy boy. Everyone who knows him says how well he looks."

Tommy's story didn't end there. At age 18, a studious young man and a good scholar, Tom began training for a professional career. He knows he owes his life to Dr. Budwig and thanks her daily in his prayers. According to his college professors, Thomas G. is showing great promise in his university work. His chosen future career, as well as his life and health, appear secure.

CARCINOMA OF THE STOMACH — When Mr. William Y. (42 years of age, husband and father of three) began suffering from chronic indigestion, he chalked it up to the stress of his job as a prominent officer of the local bank. He took over-the-counter antacid compounds to relieve his distress and ignored the problem. The condition persisted and his wife began urging him to see a doctor, but he stubbornly refused. He soon began vomiting half-digested food after eating and noticed streaks of blood in his stool after a bowel movement. Frightened and worried by these developments, Mr. Y. visited his doctor who immediately rushed him to the hospital for tests. His worst fears were realized when his doctor informed him that it appeared he had a malignant tumor growing in his digestive tract. Fortunately for Mr. Y., there was as yet no involvement of the lymph glands. (Because the lymph travels swiftly through the body, any involvement of the lymph nodes means that the malignancy can spread very quickly to other sites. In the case of lymph cancer, prognosis is extremely poor.)

Mr. Y. underwent an operation to surgically remove (excise) the cancerous growth, which appeared to be totally enclosed within its outer membrane. However, because of the possible danger of the blood stream carrying minute cancer cells to other parts of the body, Mr. Y. was placed on a program of advanced chemotherapy on an out-patient basis. He suffered all the classic side-effects of this toxic treatment, including violent vomiting and retching, progressive physical weakness, and almost complete loss of hair. The exhausted and nauseated Mr. Y. complained that the 'cure' was almost too terrible to bear.

Finally, a sympathetic friend brought Mrs. Y. some printed material which told in detail of the success of linseed oil and enriched protein in cases similar to that of her husband. The desperate wife and mother purchased some cottage cheese and a vial of raw, cold-processed, unrefined linseed oil and coaxed Mr. Y. to have it as his luncheon every day. Beginning by choking down just a few small spoonfuls daily, Mr. Y. progressed to the point where he was able to enjoy the entire amount. At this writing, Mr..Y. has returned to his employment as a bank officer and is once again able to support his family. He has completely regained his former robust health. As a preventive measure, the entire family now takes a salad of linseed oil and cottage cheese flavored with a variety of flavorful herbs daily.

OSTEOSCLEROTIC SARCOMA — When he was 16 years old, Keith O'B. was told by the Chief Surgeon of a prestigious hospital that it looked like only an amputation of his right leg could save his life. A biopsy of young Keith's tissue was taken, which verified the surgeon's initial diagnosis. He was immediately started on an intensive program of radiation treatments, but still no improvement was noted. This young high school track star said he would rather face death than lose his leg. The situation appeared hopeless. Keith's distraught parents consulted with the most eminent doctors they could locate in many areas, but all confirmed the frightening prognosis.

Only a meeting with Dr. Johanna Budwig and her words of hope stopped the planned amputation in time. After just two weeks on the Budwig formula, Keith was able to completely extend his right leg straight out for the first time in many months. A medical examination conducted two months later revealed that the swelling of Keith's involved leg had receded considerably and his blood count had returned to normal. Shortly after that, Keith's weight was stabilized and his general feeling of well-being was much improved. Within just three months of starting on the linseed oil/cottage cheese diet regimen, he was back in school. The family reports that the Budwig formula remains a part of their daily diet. The entire family, including Keith, is in excellent health.

HYPERTENSION — A harried and stressed criminal attorney of 47 years of age, Mr. Whitman W. was not surprised when his physician told him he was suffering from high blood pressure and would have to take prescribed medication for the rest of his life as he was risking collapse from a heart attack or stroke. Mr. W.'s doctor also advised him to take a vacation and take it easy in his professional life. Mr. W. laughed shortly and briefly outlined the important cases he had on his calendar that would require long days and longer nights of dedicated hard work and intense concentration. He continued working at his normal furious pace until he was faced with extreme exhaustion and could no longer ignore his health.

Mr. W. was finally forced to turn his case load over to a colleague. He checked into a renowned European health clinic and spa and prepared to take the rest he needed to renew himself. The director of this famous clinic was an advocate of linseed oil and insisted that the patients be served linseed oil and cottage cheese daily. The chef outdid himself to make the required portions tasty and used different herbs and seasonings every day. Mr. W. discovered that he looked forward to and actually relished his daily cottage cheese salad, but didn't understand just why it was 'required eating.' It was not until his blood pressure registered normal without medication that the director took him aside and explained the effects and benefits of using linseed oil with protein-rich cottage cheese. Mr. W. has incorporated this simple meal into his daily diet and now finds his tolerance to stress has been immeasurably enhanced. He no longer has hypertension and his doctor has said he has conquered the risk of suffering a sudden heart attack or paralyzing stroke.

ATHEROSCLEROSIS — A middle-aged construction worker of 50, Mr. Hank C., was told by his doctor that his serum cholesterol was registering at a very high level and he was in danger of developing an arterial blockage which could result in a stroke or serious heart attack. This nutritionally-oriented and enlightened doctor outlined the dietary changes he wanted Mr. C. to make in his eating habits and emphasized the importance of including linseed oil and cottage cheese on the menu every day. Mr. C. carried the instructions home to his wife and she immediately visited the local market, made the necessary purchases, and began serving the exact meals that the doctor had prescribed.

After two months of healthy eating, including a daily salad of cottage cheese dressed with linseed oil, the doctor was very pleased to find that Mr. C's dangerously high serum cholesterol level had been significantly lowered and pronounced him free of the imminent possibility of a blockage-induced heart seizure or sudden stroke.

BRAIN TUMOR — When Scotty A. experienced blurred vision, loss of balance and coordination, plus a complete shut-down of his bladder with the resulting pain and pressure of suppressed urine, he went to a nearby medical research center for a series of tests. The examination showed arachnoidal bleeding due to a brain tumor. (The arachnoidea is a delicate intermediate membrane which encloses the brain and spinal cord.)

Mr. A. was promptly admitted to the hospital, a catheter was fixed in place to empty his bladder continually, and chemotherapy treatment began immediately. Because of the location of the tumor, the doctors feared an operation would leave Mr. A. both paralyzed and without his mental faculties. During the course of treatment, Mr. A.'s condition worsened and his health deteriorated rapidly. His arms and legs became paralyzed and he couldn't hold any food on his stomach at all. No matter what he was fed, he vomited violently. Intravenous feeding was administered. The muscles controlling his eyes became paralyzed, leaving his eyes in an open fixed position. In order to keep the delicate eye mechanisms moistened, drops were administered around-the-clock. The medical doctors and scientists of the Research Center informed Mr. A. that he was beyond medical help. At his expressed wish, Mr. A. was discharged from the hospital and sent home to die in peace.

A Swiss friend came hurrying to his bedside bringing both comfort and hope in the form of Dr. Budwig's formula. Scotty A. was surprised to find that the few mouthfuls of the formula he was able to take stayed down. He writes: "Since I went on the Budwig regimen, the paralysis of my eyes, arms, and legs has receded daily. After only a short period of time, I was able to urinate normally. After eight weeks on the diet, I was able to walk unaided for the first time in months. My health improved so rapidly that I was soon able to return to my work part-time. Shortly after that, I was again examined at the Research Center and my reflexes were completely normal. The Budwig diet saved my life! Ten years later, I was given a thorough examination at the Center as a follow-up. My incredible recovery has been written up in many medical journals and I have become what they call a 'text-book case,' and all because of Dr. Johanna Budwig's simple diet."

FAULTY METABOLISM — A young up-and-coming career woman of 33, Miss Georgine A., had been taking thyroid medication for many years on the advice of her physician, but still found herself grossly overtired, easily irritated, and continually fighting a tendency to put on weight. This attractive young woman literally put herself on what was almost a starvation diet in an attempt to maintain a svelte figure. When she responded to what was a very real cry from her body for help and 'fell off her diet,' she gorged on saturated fats and sweets.

When this happened, she often cried herself to sleep at night and fasted the following day in an attempt to make up for what she called her 'indulgence' the day before.

What Miss. A viewed as a lack of will power and indulgence was actually an attempt by her body to stimulate her into supplying the essential fatty acids and complex carbohydrates it required for healthy metabolism. Where she went wrong was in supplying heavily saturated fats and sugary carbohydrates instead.

One day as she was eating a hasty lunch of cottage cheese at her desk, she was joined by a co-worker who was having the same little meal. The co-worker took a vial of linseed oil from her handbag and proceeded to lace her dish of cottage cheese with it. Knowing this friend to be one who never 'dieted,' Miss A. questioned her about this 'strange practice' and was thus introduced to Dr. Budwig's ideas. We are pleased to be able to tell you that Miss A. now makes one of her daily meals linseed oil and cottage cheese and says she 'never felt better' in her life. Her days of seesaw dieting are behind her; she has tremendous energy and is moving up quite steadily in her career.

THE LINSEED OIL DIET
ACCORDING TO DR. JOHANNA BUDWIG

Dr. Budwig is very strict when prescribing nutritional therapy for her patients. For those of you who are in real need of this information, but unable to make a trip to Germany, we are providing an examination of Dr. Budwig's methods, as experienced by Jane D., a close family friend well-known to some of my European relatives.

To my knowledge, this is the first time this important information has been brought to the attention of the American public. I know first-hand of the documented successes Dr. Budwig has achieved in treating her patients, including some who were considered terminally ill by the orthodox medical community. However, it is not the intent of the author to persuade anyone to discontinue medical treatment.

FOR THE SERIOUSLY ILL

Because Janie D. was unable to keep food down, her treatment started with linseed oil (4 to 8.5 ounces) enemas of this miracle oil. After a few days on the enema regimen, Jane was taking 8 ounces of freshly ground linseed (flaxseed) mixed with raw honey,* the first food she had taken by mouth in some time. Jane was able to tolerate this mixture surprisingly easily. *(Note: The consumption of honey is not advised for diabetics. Because honey is an integral part of the diet Janie herself followed, diabetics are especially warned against taking honey [where indicated], until and unless the regimen is first approved and regulated by a doctor.)

According to Dr. Budwig herself, any seriously (or even moderately) ill person will benefit by taking ground linseed and honey. Jane was given this mixture for a few days until her digestion improved and she began to feel better. She was also allowed freshly made fruit juices *without any sugar.* Especially recommended are fresh vegetable juices (carrot or celery), plus apple juice. (If prepared juices are purchased, make sure there are no preservatives or chemical additives of any kind. If you have a good juicer, it's best to prepare your own juices at home so that you know exactly what's in them.)

Jane was told that it was very important that she take a warm drink three times daily. Herbal teas (such as peppermint or rose hips), are excellent and may be sweetened slightly with honey. Sugar is expressly forbidden. Grape juice can be used alone, or to sweeten other juices, when necessary. A small amount of regular tea may be taken in the morning (a.m. only).

THE ALTERNATIVE — OATMEAL MASH

Jane was soon able to tolerate the pure ground linseeds with honey mixture very well, but her family had a healthy alternative to fall back on when she was feeling particularly weak. Here's how Janie's family fixed the Oatmeal Mash, in accordance with Dr. Budwig's teaching:

Put 3 tablespoons of uncooked oatmeal in 4-6 ounces of cold water and bring to a boil. Add to this soft mash, 3 tablespoons of freshly ground linseed (flaxseed). Simmer briefly and allow to stand over very low heat for ten minutes. Remove the linseed mash from heat and strain. A little milk may be added if desired, which also benefits the digestion. This mixture is of high nutritive value.

To vary the taste of the linseed/oatmeal mash, Jane's family prepared it with several different healthy nutrients. Janie's favorites additions were: (1) Mix ¼ cup fresh carrot juice into the hot mash and take immediately. Carrot juice should be ingested as soon as it is prepared and not allowed to stand, or (2) You may stir in ¼ cup fresh orange juice, or (3) Stir in ¼ cup grape juice (red or white), or (4) Stir in 2 tablespoons of very finely grated apple.

THE STANDARD LINSEED OIL REGIMEN:

After a few days on the cleansing and building regimens as given in detail above, the next step for Jane was to proceed to the standard dietary program. Because of Janie's long-standing illness and seriously weakened condition, the family put her on the following hour-by-hour very strict nutritional program, highly recommended by a friend who was treated by Dr. Budwig:

At 7:00 am: On an empty stomach, Janie took 2-4 ounces of sauerkraut juice. Note: Sauerkraut juice has a high lactic acid content which enhances fat permeation, reduces congestion, and facilitates fat metabolism, thereby cleansing and flushing out blockages. It also aids the digestive process. Even those with a sensitive stomach benefit from the lactic acid content of sauerkraut juice and soon find that even raw vegetables are easily tolerated.

At 8:00 am: Before eating breakfast, Jane had 4-6 ounces of warm herb (or regular) tea. Next, she especially enjoyed the breakfast 'muesli' the family prepared for her, as follows: In a deep dish, layer in bowl in order given: (1) 3-4 tablespoons freshly ground linseed (flaxseed). (2) Add any fresh fruit in season (sliced or diced), and/or fresh fruit juice (without sugar or chemical additives), (3) Optional: Add a layer of any kind of ground nuts (except peanuts), (4) To 3-4 ounces of low-fat cottage cheese, add 1 teaspoon honey, 1-2 tablespoons linseed oil, 3 tablespoons raw milk, and blend together. It is important to use a blender or electric mixer so that the mixture becomes completely homogenized. (Add a little additional milk if necessary). Then, (5) Layer the cottage cheese/linseed oil mixture over the other ingredients in the bowl. For variety, you may add any of the following to the cottage cheese mixture: Bananas, lemon juice, orange juice (mixed 2 to 1), carob powder, coconut (unsweetened), vanilla, cinnamon, and so on. (We remind you again that diabetics should avoid the use of honey, unless specifically permitted its use by their doctor.)

Between 10 am to 11 am: As a mid-morning pick-me-up, Janie had 4-6 ounces fresh carrot juice. One half hour later, she choose from a selection of either radish juice, nettle juice (with lemon), celery juice or beet juice (mixed with apple juice).

12 noon (lunch): Just before lunch, Jane took 1 tablespoon freshly ground linseed (flaxseed) mixed with honey and 4-6 ounces of grape juice.

After fifteen minutes (12:15 pm): The first course of Janie's noon meal was a salad consisting of: Dandelion greens, watercress, celery tops, radish, sauerkraut, freshly ground horseradish (not made with vinegar), and green bell peppers. This delicious salad was topped with a mayonnaise made from cottage cheese, linseed oil, milk, fresh lemon, a little salt, mustard, pickles, garlic, plus fresh (or dried) herbs to taste, whipped to a creamy consistency in a blender.

At 12:30 pm: For the second 'course,' of her health-building luncheon, Jane was served a tasty bowl of fresh vegetables (choose your favorites) simmered in a little water with herbs, curry powder, or a little linseed oil for rich flavor. (This vegetable broth may also be seasoned separately with yeast flakes or bouillon.) Along with her veggies, Janie sometimes had buckwheat (cooked as for rice), brown rice, potatoes boiled in the jacket, or fresh mashed potatoes (made with

155

a little milk and linseed oil). As Janie began to feel better, she craved a sweet. Her favorite desert was the layered cottage cheese/linseed oil fruit salad described above, with a little extra honey and natural vanilla added.

At 3:00 pm: Janie's mid-afternoon pick-me-up was one tablespoon of freshly ground linseed (flaxseed) with honey and 4-6 ounces of grape juice (unsweetened), or fresh pineapple juice.

At 3:30 pm: After a half an hour, she had an additional one to three tablespoons freshly ground linseed (flaxseed) with honey and three glasses (6 to 18 ounces total) of fresh cherry or blackberry juice.

At 6:00 pm: Janie's light evening meal consisted of one cup (6 ounces) of soup made of buckwheat cooked in vegetable broth, seasoned with a little linseed oil for good flavor and 1 teaspoon yeast flakes.

At 8:30 pm: Before she retired, Janie enjoyed 4-6 ounces grape juice with 1 tablespoon honey added.

I am very pleased to be able to report that Janie D. improved tremendously on this special diet. At the end of just two weeks on the complete program, her energy levels were so repaired that she was fussing at her family because she wanted to get out of bed and do things.

Today, just seven months later, Janie is again caring for her husband, her three children, and her household single-handed. Someone meeting this radiant woman for the first time wouldn't recognize her as the frail degenerated person she was less than a year ago! You'd better believe that Janie has the whole family enjoying a portion of cottage cheese dressed with linseed oil every day.

Note: It may seem as if this around-the-clock dietary program is overdone, but I assure you that run-down and debilitated individuals benefit immeasureably by eating the recommended foods as specified. The seriously (or even moderately) ill person needs to eat more often to rebuild and strengthen the body.

*Freshly ground linseed (flaxseed) and honey is an important part of the recommended diet. This nutritional supplement is sold already prepared abroad under the name of *Linomel,* but is not yet available in the U.S. However, the preparation can be made at home by purchasing whole linseeds (flaxseed) and putting them through a nut grinder before mixing the crushed seeds with raw honey. We stress (again) that diabetics should not take honey except on the approval of a doctor.

A SIMPLE SUGGESTION

It's hard to believe that simply supplying the body with a daily dose (one tablespoon) of raw, cold-processed, unrefined, virgin linseed oil with the good quality protein present in (one-half cup) low-fat cottage cheese can make such a vital difference in health, but the benefits of incorporating this simple meal into the diet are well documented and backed by sound research. The essential fatty acids (linoleic, linolenic) that the body requires for healthy functioning and efficient metabolism of lipids (fats) are present in natural abundance in this ancient botanical, recently rediscovered.

As you have read in the foregoing material, scientists all over the world are quite rightly singing the praises of *Linum usitatissimum:* linseed oil. You just might want to consider the possible health benefits of adding a linseed oil dressed, herb flavored, low-fat cottage cheese salad to your daily menu. Judging by the unprecedented results achieved in research, it must be said that dietary linseed oil has to be an extremely powerful natural preventive and unparalleled therapeutic treatment as well.

It always pleasures us to bring you important news of a medicinal or botanical nature. Correctly produced (raw, cold-processed, unrefined, virgin) linseed oil is difficult, but not impossible to obtain in the United States. Dr. Budwig urges obtaining a brand produced to retain all its vital health-promoting properties. Several health companies have raw linseed oil but Dr. Budwig suggests you check to make sure it is the unrefined virgin linseed oil before making a purchase.

Chapter VII

The Dietary Delights of Linseed Oil

How To Enjoy The Miracle Fat

THE BASIC FORMULA

As a dietary supplement, I personally take 1 or 2 tablespoons of cold-processed, unrefined virgin linseed oil mixed with ½ to 1 cup of low-fat cottage cheese every day. Because of all the very strong evidence, it seems to me that this is the best 'preventive medicine' in the world to ward off the degenerative diseases.

HOW TO PREPARE A LINSEED OIL & COTTAGE CHEESE SALAD

To the basic formula given above, we add herbs, raw vegetables, or fruits to taste, exactly as recommended by Dr. Johanna Budwig. We mince the herbs finely (or crumble dried herbs), grate raw vegetables, dice or chop fruits, and whirl in a blender until well mixed. The use of a blender is strongly recommended to insure that the oil permeates the cottage cheese completely and that the salad is well-flavored with your favorite additions.

The use of a different variety of flavorings is recommended so as not to tire of this healthy mixture. Garlic and onions are very popular health-promoting additions. Try finely grated cucumbers and radishes with some chopped tomatoes and a crumbling of dill. A combination of grated carrots and minced onions is both tasty and healthy.

For a sensational naturally sweet salad, coarsely chop a tart-sweet apple, add a small handful of raisins, a sprinkling of cinnamon, and a dollop of (raw) honey to taste.

The idea is to experiment by adding your own favorite herbs, vegetables, and fruits to the basic linseed oil and cottage cheese formula to provide variety.

MY FAVORITE BREAKFAST 'MUESLI' (MIXTURE)

Before eating this delightful breakfast 'muesli,' we take a cup (4-6 ounces) of warm herb (or regular) tea, in accordance with the standard regimen.

Here's how we prepare the 'muesli.' In a deep bowl, layer (do not blend together) in order given: (1) 1 to 2 tablespoons freshly ground linseed blended with a little honey (optional). (2) Add any fresh fruit in season (sliced or diced), and/or canned fruits or juices (without sugar or chemical additives), (3) Optional: Add a layer of any kind of ground nuts (except peanuts), (4) Prepare *cream topping*, as follows: To 3-4 ounces of low-fat cottage cheese, add 1 teaspoon honey, 1 to 2 tablespoons linseed oil, 3 tablespoons low-fat milk, and blend together. (It is important to use a blender or electric mixer so that the mixture becomes completely homogenized. Add a little additional milk if necessary).

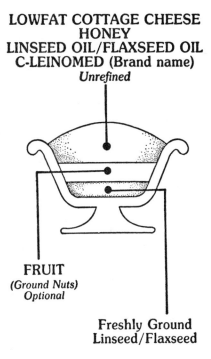

LOWFAT COTTAGE CHEESE
HONEY
LINSEED OIL/FLAXSEED OIL
C-LEINOMED (Brand name)
Unrefined

FRUIT
(Ground Nuts)
Optional

Freshly Ground
Linseed/Flaxseed

Then, (5) Spoon the cream topping mixture over the other ingredients in the bowl. Top with a sprinkling of nuts, chopped fruits, spices, or herbs.

For variety, we may add just about anything we like to the linseed oil/cottage cheese cream topping. Try bananas, lemon juice and orange juice (mixed 2 to 1), your favorite fruit juice, carob powder, coconut (unsweetened), vanilla, cinnamon, and on and on.

My wife and I enjoy this special 'muesli' every day. Please don't think you can eat it only for breakfast; it often serves as a light luncheon or dinner for us. I have introduced our friends to this delightful combination and we've had many favorable comments, especially pertaining to an incredible rush of sustained energy and easy weight loss.

One of my favorite people is a rather elderly gentleman (age 75) who lives nearby. Over the last few years, I have watched him with a great deal of sadness as he became frail and stooped. He got around painfully by supporting himself with a stout cane and it was apparent that he suffered greatly from arthritis. I tried tactfully to advise him on the importance of eating correctly, but he always laughed and wouldn't listen to any serious conversation on the subject of his health.

We were chatting a few months ago about inconsequential things when my wife called out the window to tell me that lunch was ready. I coaxed him into joining us and introduced him to the 'muesli.' He devoured a whole heaping dishful with obvious pleasure. Since that time, I know for a fact that he fixes himself a cottage cheese salad generously laced with this liquid sunshine every day. His improvement has been gradual, but he is improving. On many days, he leaves his stick at home because he really doesn't need it anymore. His formerly sick and waxy complexion has become pink with the glow of health and he continually expresses his gratitude for the increased well-being he is experiencing.

DRESSINGS FOR SALAD GREENS & RAW VEGETABLES

We eat a lot of salads fixed with a variety of greens (spinach is a particular favorite) and slivered raw vegetables. I like variety, so we use many different homemade dressings. Here's a few suggestions to get you started. Beginning with the basic blend of 1 tablespoon of cold-processed, unrefined linseed oil mixed with ½ to 1 cup of low-fat cottage cheese, try the following mixtures: *Creamy Italian* — Add vinegar and Italian herbs to taste. This is not only delicious on crisp greens, but also delightful as a dip for raw vegetables. *Thousand Island* — Add a little lemon juice, a little tomato juice, chopped hard boiled egg, and dill pickle. You may add honey to taste if you like this dressing slightly sweet. *Poppyseed Sweet & Sour* — Add honey for the sweet and lemon juice for the sour. Spark with a little dijon mustard, sprinkle in a generous amount of poppyseeds and enjoy. Wonderful on both a fresh fruit salad or the traditional greens. *Russian Dressing* — Add honey and lemon juice (as above), plus tomato juice (to taste). *Green Goddess* — Mince cucumbers, spinach leaves, and a little parsley. Whirl into the basic mixture and season with dill. *Hot Stuff* — Add cayenne pepper, minced chile peppers, a finely diced red bell pepper, minced onion, and blend well. Refrigerate for at least one hour to allow the flavors to meld. A real party-pickup when served with crisp raw vegetables for dipping.

THE BREAD SPREADS

Linseed Oil Butter — Many health-food stores offer sesame butter, but linseed oil butter is healthier and tastes better, to my way of thinking. The recipe follows: First, put 100 grams of crude linseed oil in the freezer to chill thoroughly. Then gently heat 8 ounces of coconut oil to boiling. (Note: Natural coconut oil is available in most health food stores.) Add a mashed clove of garlic and a medium onion cut in quarters to the simmering coconut oil. When the garlic and onions turn transparent (but before they brown), remove them with a slotted spoon and discard. Allow the melted coconut oil to cool off, but before it firms up, pour it into the chilled linseed oil. Blend thoroughly and pop your linseed oil butter back into the freezer to harden.

161

The garlic and onions add the sulphur the body needs to efficiently protect and process the essential fatty acids present in the linseed oil, so they are important additions. If you wish, you may substitute oats, peppers, or buckwheat in the recipe to provide the organic sulphur, but the resulting butter will be very bland. In either case, you'll find your linseed oil butter spreads nicely and is nutritionally correct. It is many times better than butter from the dairy and at least a thousand times better for you than the artificially hardened chemically saturated mess of fat known as margarine.

Mayonnaise — For a quick and nutritious bread-spread, add a dab of milk to the basic mixture, season with a spicy salt-free blend of powdered herbs (the supermarket has several good ones), and homogenize completely in a blender. (One of my all-time favorite additions to this mayonnaise is horseradish, freshly grated if possible.)

THE MAIN MEAL

Any meal should begin with a portion of raw, uncooked foods. We like to start off with a mixed green and raw vegetable salad topped with one of the dressing recipes given earlier. We always add some shredded carrots in our salads for their rich content of beta-carotene. Or we sometimes begin the meal with a slice of melon or other fresh fruit. Next, we have a side dish of the basic linseed oil/cottage cheese mixture, well flavored with our favorite additions.

We often have a bowl of good homemade soup, such as lentil, barley, or pea, for some high-quality vegetable protein. Adding a fluffy baked potato alongside makes the meal particularly satisfying. We sometimes enjoy potatoes with linseed oil butter and powdered herbs and spices, but my personal favorite is fixed this way: I cut the hot potato in half (the long way); top it with a scoop of low-fat cottage cheese; drizzle on some golden linseed oil; add some raw sweet onion (finely minced), and then fork the topping mixture all through the tender meat of the potato. A sprinkling of paprika on top, and the common old spud is transformed into an epicurean delight.

THE SWEET FINALE

I can't help it. I have to finish off a meal with a bite of something sweet, but I don't have to feel guilty about it when that something sweet begins with the basic linseed oil and cottage cheese mixture. It's easy to add a handful of berries in season (or any other of Mother Nature's sweet fruits), a spoonful of honey (or a dab of maple syrup, sensational with minced apple), and some vanilla (cinnamon, nutmeg, cloves, allspice, mint). Stir in any chopped nuts (except peanuts) for a family delight — or top with some slivered almonds for an elegant 'company' dessert.

A FINAL NOTE

The beauty of it is that the golden healing nutrition of linseed oil and the sulphur-based proteins of low-fat cottage cheese which comprise the basic mixture are bland enough alone to lend themselves to just about any combination of flavors that you can come up with. The possibilities are virtually unlimited. Let your imagination be your guide. Have fun with it by providing variety — and let the dietary delights of this healthful healing combination of the essential fatty acids and quality proteins insure you and your family of vibrant health and vitality forever.

PROCEED WITH CAUTION — My enthusiasm for the nutritional gold of virgin linseed oil must be toned down with a word of advice. This liquid sunshine is incredibly rich in the essential fats which, as we have discovered to our sorrow, are usually deficient in the American diet. For this reason, those new to this way of eating should make haste slowly so as not to shock a system accustomed to chemically altered and refined foods. It is best to begin with only a scant teaspoon of linseed oil blended into one-half to one cup of low-fat cottage cheese daily for a period of a few days to allow your body to adjust. And I remind you again that diabetics should not use honey, except with permission of their doctor.

DR. BUDWIG'S 4-WEEK ANTI-CANCER MENU

How can you put flaxseed and flaxseed oil to work for you? We asked Dr. Budwig that, and she replied with four weeks of suggested menus. For a brush-up on flaxseed and its unique health benefits, turn back to chapter 6.

*For ground flaxseed - see recipe on page 159.
**For basic mayonnaise - see recipe on page 162.
***For linseed oil butter - see recipe on page 161.

DAY 1:

Morning: Muesli: cover 2 tablespoons of ground flaxseed* with a layer of finely-chopped banana. Pour on a little unsweetened black currant juice. Over that, spoon low-fat cottage cheese and linseed oil with honey.

Rye bread with cheese and raw vegetables.

Noon: Vegetable soup, boiled with celery and carrots. Cook the vegetables, then puree them with a tomato and a little broth. Return mixture to broth and season with yeast extract and an herbal salt mixture.

Boiled potatoes in their jackets, lowfat cottage cheese and linseed oil butter*** (season with caraway seeds). Serve with pickled cucumbers, tomato and a mixed green salad.

Dessert: one orange.

Evening: Unsweetened buckwheat pudding with naturally-sweetened or unsweetened blueberry juice.

Sandwiches made with rye bread: nothing salty.

DAY 2:

Morning: 2 tablespoons ground flaxseed*, finely chopped figs and dates combined with pureed apples as a fruit layer. Pour over low-fat cottage cheese and linseed oil and honey.

Noon: Raw vegetable platter: radish, carrots, parsley, pickled cucumbers, and apple puree.

Boiled potatoes in their jackets and spinach, sparsely sprinkled with linseed oil butter***.

Dessert: lowfat cottage cheese with linseed oil and honey. Mix and sprinkle with grated coconut.

Evening: Peppermint tea with honey.

Mixture of raw vegetables sprinkled with linseed oil.

Slice of rye bread or toast.

DAY 3:

Morning: 2 tablespoons ground flaxseed* mixed with finely cut orange slices or dates. Over that, lowfat cottage cheese with linseed oil and honey, generously sprinkled with pistachios.

Noon: Green salad with ample amount of mayonnaise** made of lowfat cottage cheese, linseed oil and lemon juice.

Long grain rice with linseed oil and honey.

Dessert: Pureed raw apples with raisins, presoftened in grape juice.

Evening: Rice pudding with long-grain rice, sweetened with honey and covered mildly with linseed oil.

Canapes: small vegetable sandwiches.

DAY 4:

Morning: Ground flaxseed*, pureed apples, lowfat cottage cheese and linseed oil, topped with grated coconut.

Noon: Lentil soup with potatoes, well-smeared with linseed oil, seasoned with yeast extract, herbs and dill.

165

Dessert: lowfat cottage cheese and linseed oil with honey, served over fruit salad.

Evening: Soybean flakes (2 tablespoons), with hot milk and pureed hazelnuts. Serve with canapes.

DAY 5:

Morning: Layer ground flaxseed*, finely chopped orange, lowfat cottage cheese and linseed oil with honey, unsweetened cocoa powder, pistachio nuts.

Noon: Green salad with linseed-lemon-cottage cheese mayonnaise**; garnished with cucumbers and chives.

Cauliflower, potatoes boiled in jackets, hot tomato sauce or salsa with poached eggs.

Dessert: melons; cantaloupe if possible.

Evening: Buckwheat cooked during the morning, cooled to a firm pudding and cut into slices. Pureed apples and raisins.

Canapes if needed.

DAY 6:

Morning: Layered ground flaxseed*, pureed apples, chopped figs mixed with a little blueberry juice; lowfat cottage cheese with linseed oil and honey.

Noon: Raw vegetable platter with radish, carrots with pureed apples, pickled vegetable, cucumber. Boiled potatoes, small-cut herring, diced cucumbers, special mayonnaise**.

Dessert: fruit.

Evening: Soybean flakes and small orange pieces with hot milk poured over. Canapes, if needed.

DAY 7:

Morning: Layered ground flaxseed* with minced apples,

pears and grapes; lowfat cottage cheese, linseed oil and honey.

Noon: Vegetable broth with raw pureed celery, tofu or yeast extract, dill and a generous dollop of linseed oil.

Boiled potatoes in their jackets with celery slices, baked in linseed oil butter***. Belgian endive salad.

Dessert: Lowfat cottage cheese with linseed oil, honey and unsweetened cocoa powder, walnuts or hazelnuts.

Evening: Long-grain rice, sweetened with honey, served with unsweetened blueberry juice. Canapes if needed.

DAY 8:

Morning: Layered ground flaxseed*, cottage cheese with linseed oil and honey; walnuts, and orange slices.

Noon: Raw vegetable platter: radish, green salad, tomatoes. Boiled potatoes, steamed vegetables (cucumbers and tomatoes) with linseed oil butter***.

Dessert: cottage cheese, linseed oil and honey with bananas.

Evening: Vegetable broth, seasoned to taste. Put pureed boiled vegetables into broth, dab with linseed oil butter***, and slowly cook 2 tablespoons of barley in the broth. Canapes if needed.

DAY 9:

Morning: Layered ground flaxseed*, raisins soaked in currant juice, mixed with pureed apples; Lowfat cottage cheese with linseed oil, honey and coconut flakes.

Noon: Broth from boiled long-grain rice, seasoned with curry and linseed oil. Serve in cups.

Long-grain rice with linseed oil butter***, tossed with mushrooms and tomatoes.

Dessert: slice of rye bread, spread with sweet butter, covered with cheese and baked, garnished with tomato.

Evening: Soy flakes soaked with hot, thinned juice.

Canapes.

DAY 10:

Morning: Layered ground flaxseed* with pureed apple, cottage cheese, linseed oil, honey and almond puree (1 teaspoon).

Noon: Raw vegetable platter: radish, carrots with pureed apples, parsley and a pickled vegetable.

Boiled potatoes with lowfat cottage cheese and linseed oil, mixed with raw bell pepper or caraway seeds.

Dessert: 1 cup buttermilk.

Evening: Peppermint tea with honey. Small sandwiches made of cheese and pickled cucumbers.

DAY 11:

Morning: Layered ground flaxseed, cottage cheese, honey, poppyseed oil (1 tablespoon). Over that, pureed apples and a generous sprinkling of poppyseeds.

Noon: Broth boiled with cauliflower, serve with raw pureed tomatoes and milk. Dab well with linseed oil butter***, season heartily with paprika. (Makes a thickened soup with small cauliflower chunks.)

Evening: Buckwheat pudding with natural, unsweetened juice. Canapes.

DAY 12:

Morning: Layered ground flaxseed* with minced orange, cottage cheese, linseed oil and honey and unsweetened cocoa mixed with ground nuts.

Noon: Raw vegetable platter. (No mayonnaise or dressing.)

Potato salad with boiled egg, made with special mayonnaise**.

Dessert: small pieces of apple and pineapple, served over low-fat cottage cheese with linseed oil and honey. Season with a sprinkling of curry powder.

Evening: Long-grain whole rice, boiled. Dab well with linseed oil butter***. Serve with raw, pureed apples with unsweetened apple juice and raisins.

DAY 13:

Morning: Ground flaxseed* layered with minced pears and a few raisins, cottage cheese and linseed oil with honey and almonds.

Noon: Clear vegetable broth made from steamed beans.

Well-seasoned beans, covered with linseed oil butter***. After removing beans from steamer, season leftover liquid with linseed oil butter*** and eat as broth.

Boiled potatoes in their jackets. French green beans spread with linseed oil butter***.

Dessert: cottage cheese with linseed oil and honey served over fruit salad.

Evening: Rose-hip tea with honey. Canapes made of raw spreads (pureed cucumbers, tomatoes and pickles).

DAY 14:

Morning: Ground flaxseed* layered with minced figs, apple puree, cottage cheese, linseed oil and honey, lemons and orange juice.

Noon: Lettuce or green salad, garnished with lemon and linseed oil.

Boiled potatoes, cottage cheese with linseed oil and chopped pickles. Serve with a small amount of pickled vegetables.

Dessert: melons or other fruit.

Evening: Rolled oats, dry, soaked with hot almond milk. (to prepare, mix several tablespoons almond puree with water, added gradually until milky. Sweeten with honey.

DAY 15:

Morning: Layered ground flaxseed* with raisins pre-softened in white grape juice, cottage cheese, linseed oil, honey. Serve with a cheese sandwich.

Noon: Raw vegetable platter: grated carrots, pureed apples, dressed with a tablespoon of almond puree. Sprinkle with orange juice.

Grated kohlrabi with a little almond puree.

Potato pancakes baked in linseed oil. (to prepare: thicken a portion of mashed potatoes with soy flour, add pureed onion and season with herbal salt. Serve with pureed apples.)

Eggs prepared as desired.

Evening: Small sandwiches made with pickles, cream cheese, pickled cauliflower and carrots.

DAY 16:

Morning: Ground flaxseed* layered with cottage cheese, linseed oil, honey, ground almonds soaked in grape juice.

Canapes with Camembert cheese.

Noon: Soup made with brussels sprout water, seasoned with linseed oil butter***, herbal salt and paprika. Serve with raw, pureed tomatoes, carrots and celery.

Potatoes in their jackets, brussels sprouts with linseed oil butter***.

Dessert: cottage cheese, linseed oil and honey over tangerine pieces.

Evening: Small sandwiches made with tomatoes, radish, cream cheese and pickles.

DAY 17:

Morning: Ground flaxseed* layered with pureed walnuts. Over that, cottage cheese, linseed oil and honey.

Noon: Raw vegetable platter: beets, grated finely with walnut oil and grated apple dressing. The beets must be allowed to stand at least two hours to soften.

Millet paste, seasoned with herbal salt and spread with linseed oil butter***, served with paprika sauce. (to make: puree 1 onion, 2 tomatoes, 2 tablespoons linseed oil butter***. Heat briefly, season with herbal salt and pour over millet.)

Dice quinces, cooked till soft, sweetened with honey, linseed oil and quince juice mixture.

Evening: Soup made with broth from long-grain rice, seasoned with curry and covered with linseed oil butter***. Serve with small cream cheese and tomato sandwiches.

DAY 18:

Morning: Ground flaxseed* layered with cottage cheese, linseed oil, honey and poppyseed oil. Sprinkle with poppyseed and wet with a little juice.

Small cheese sandwiches.

Noon: Lentil soup boiled with leeks, seasoned with linseed oil butter***. Serve with pureed leeks, paprika, tofu and herbal salt.

Dessert: a glass of white grape juice.

Evening: Long-grain rice sweetened with honey, dabbed with sweet butter. Serve with pureed apples and raisins softened in currant juice.

DAY 19:

Morning: Ground flaxseed* layered with cottage cheese, linseed oil and honey. Mix a generous amount of minced fresh pineapple into the cottage cheese and serve immediately.

Noon: Soup made from broth of lima and kidney beans, seasoned with herbal salt, sweet butter and yeast extract. Served with the cooked beans, raw tomatoes and carrots.

Boiled potatoes in their jackets with green beans spread with sweet butter.

Dessert: low-fat cottage cheese with linseed oil, honey and pineapple.

Evening: Unsweetened hot cocoa. Canapes with cream cheese, caraway seeds, parsley and sliced cucumbers.

DAY 20:

Morning: Ground flaxseed* layered with diced pears, cottage cheese, linseed oil, honey and chopped pistachios.

Noon: Soup cooked with celery leaves, carrots and leeks. Add pureed vegetables to the broth, season with tofu and linseed oil butter***.

Boil potatoes in their jackets, serve with cottage

cheese and linseed oil mixed with pureed caraway or parsley.

Dessert: stuffed dates. Split open nicely formed dates, remove the seeds and stuff with walnuts, Brazil or pistachio nuts.

Evening: Buckwheat pudding with unsweetened blueberry juice. Canapes with linseed oil butter*** and cream cheese.

DAY 21:

Morning: Ground flaxseed* layered with pureed apples and juice-soaked raisins; cottage cheese, linseed oil and honey.

Noon: Belgian endive salad with special mayonnaise** seasoned with pickles and lemon.

Long-grain rice spread with linseed oil butter*** add pureed tomatoes and steamed bell peppers.

Evening: Soy flakes soaked in hot milk, with hazelnut puree. Small finger sandwiches (use Party Rye bread) made with tomato, radish and cucumber.

DAY 22:

Morning: Ground flaxseed layered with cottage cheese, linseed oil and honey, plus a tablespoon of poppyseed oil and a sprinkling of poppyseeds.

Noon: Raw vegetable platter: kohlrabi with almond puree, parsley, small cucumber, beet and walnut oil dressing.

Dessert: Cottage cheese, linseed oil, honey with rose-hip puree.

Evening: Buckwheat pudding served with raw, pureed apples. Season with anise.

DAY 23:

Morning: Ground flaxseed* mixed with a generous amount of blueberry juice. Over that, spoon cottage cheese, linseed oil and honey.

Noon: Kale stew, covered with linseed oil butter***. Serve with a baked celery slice.

Dessert: Lowfat cottage cheese, linseed oil and honey garnished with walnuts.

Evening: Long grain rice soup with milk, sweetened with honey. Canapes made of linseed oil butter***, cream cheese, caraway seeds and parsley.

DAY 24:

Morning: Ground flaxseed* layered with minced tangerines, lowfat cottage cheese and linseed oil honey pureed with one or two tangerines.

Noon: Warm soup made from vegetable water with raw, pureed tomatoes and carrots.

Boiled potatoes in their jackets; Lowfat cottage cheese and linseed oil with parsley or caraway seeds.

Dessert: fruit salad with walnut oil. (no cottage cheese.)

Evening: Canapes made with cheese, radish and cucumbers.

DAY 25:

Morning: Ground flaxseed* with lowfat cottage cheese, linseed oil, honey served with grated coconut and coconut milk.

Noon: Lentil soup with uncooked sauerkraut, spread with linseed oil butter***.

Dessert: a glass of unsweetened fruit juice.

Evening: Canapes with cream cheese and caraway or Camembert cheese and paprika.

DAY 26:

Morning: Ground flaxseed* layered with cottage cheese, linseed oil, honey and diced fresh pineapple. Bread with Edam cheese and Swiss cheese.

Noon: Raw vegetable platter with kohlrabi, carrots, pickled vegetables. Cauliflower with linseed oil butter***. Boiled potatoes in their jackets.

Dessert: cottage cheese, linseed oil, honey and banana.

Evening: Cup of soup made from cauliflower broth: Puree lunch leftovers with hand mixer, serve warm with sandwiches made from pickles, tomato and cream cheese.

DAY 27:

Morning: Ground flaxseed* layered with diced pears, topped with special mayonnaise**.

Noon: Brussels sprouts spread with linseed oil butter***.

Boiled potatoes in their jackets.

One Banana.

Evening: Soy flakes soaked with hot milk, served with almond puree.

Canapes with cheese or mushroom paste.

DAY 28:

Morning: Ground flaxseed*, pureed apples and juice-soaked raisins; cottage cheese, linseed oil, honey, a sprinkling of fruit juice.

Noon: Endive salad with linseed oil mayonnaise** and pickles.

Buckwheat and mushrooms.

Canapes made from Swiss and American cheeses.

Evening: Leftovers from noon meal, pureed and heated as soup. Cream cheese canapes with radish.

Chapter VIII

Golden Bee Pollen Is Real 'Health Insurance'

A Potent Cancer Preventive and Much More

In ancient China, natural healers were paid a monthly stipend to watch over a family. Their task was to keep all the family members well. These early physicians were regularly consulted on all matters pertaining to health, prescribed herbal preventives, scolded when an ill-advised action threatened the well being of one in their care, and generally practiced a very effective form of preventive medicine. If an individual in their charge fell ill, the monthly fee was not paid by the family until that person was returned to robust and glowing health. I call that true 'health insurance!' In direct contrast, consider that our modern doctors are not paid until we develop a sickness. But in the highly cultured and advanced civilization of China centuries ago, the physicians had a very real incentive to practice good preventive medicine. That miracle food from the beehive, bee pollen, is amazingly effective preventive medicine and it doesn't require a doctor's prescription either!

BEE POLLEN IS SUPERIOR PREVENTIVE MEDICINE — As did the physicians of old, the natural healers of today call bee pollen a very effective form of 'health insurance.' One of the most interesting things about bee pollen is that it *cannot*

176

be synthesized in a laboratory. Oh yes, bee pollen contains all the vitamins, minerals, amino acids (proteins), hormones, enzymes, carbohydrates, essential fatty acids, and trace elements known to be needed in human nutrition. But, as if that were not enough, Mother Nature (personified by the bee) adds a mysterious extra that has so far defied scientific analysis. In fact, some researchers believe it's this mysterious unidentifiable extra constituent which makes bee pollen the powerhouse nutrition that it is. It's important to note here that pollen collected mechanically directly from plants (sometimes called 'flower pollen') without the intervention of the bee is without this important extra factor.

Another one of nature's little mysteries is the fact that bee pollen contains a live electric charge. Dr. Eric H. Erickson, of the University of Wisconsin's Entomology Department, reports that when the worker bees leave the hive, they have a slightly negative or neutral electrical charge. But, upon returning to the hive with their pollen baskets loaded, the same bees register a positive charge of electricity as great as 1.5 volts. The live energized bee pollen they carry is also electrically charged.

Just what is this incredible natural substance? Pollen is the live male spore of all botanicals and is necessary for fertilization and growth of the species. Each microscopically tiny speck of this golden dust has the ability to reproduce. Bees unerringly select only the most powerful and potent pollens as food for the hive, another reason why bee pollen is superior to mechanically-collected pollen. Although the adult worker bees subsist on honey, the tiny larvae are fed bee pollen to insure a good start in life.

Because the Queen begins life as a larva exactly like any other bee destined to become a worker, it is an indisputable fact that her exclusive diet of royal jelly (produced from bee pollen) is what causes her to become a creature far superior to the workers of the hive. The theory that bee pollen contains a rejuvenating, health-promoting, and life-extending force is based on the fact that the Queen bee alone lives for five or six *years* on her royal diet of royal jelly (which the bees manufacture from pollen), while the worker bees who eat only honey live for merely a matter of weeks.

EXAMINING THE EVIDENCE

INCREASING THE LIFE SPAN - Who says so? The Queen bee, Noel Johnson (the 95-year old Gold Medal marathon runner- born in 1899), and U.S. President Ronald Reagan (born in 1911, now age 83, and a well-publicized proponent of bee pollen), are not the only ones who acknowledge the power of pollen to extend life expectancy beyond the norm.

The countries behind the Iron Curtain have published considerable research on the beneficial effects of this near-perfect food. Professor Dr. Nikolai V. Tsitsin, U.S.S.R. botanist and biologist, investigated the lifestyle of the centenarians past 125 years of age living in the Caucasus mountains of upper Russia. He reported that many were beekeepers and the villagers all ate the sticky residue found on the bottom of the hives as one of their principal foods.

On analyzing this mass, Tsitsin found it to be almost pure bee pollen. After intensive research, he determined that including bee pollen in their regular diet was responsible in a large part for the incredible age these people attained. Tsitsin was also impressed with the quality of their lives in that all these people were actively working and in singularly good health in spite of their advanced age.

Working independently, the same conclusions were reached by other U.S.S.R. scientists as well. Dr. Naum P. Yoirich of the Soviet Academy summarizes his research in these words, "Bee pollen is one of the original treasure-houses of nutrition and medicine. *Long lives are attained by bee pollen users.* It contains every important substance necessary to life."

Perhaps even more important for those of us discovering bee pollen late in life is the statement made by the Far East Institute of the Soviet Union in Vladivostok. These scientists concluded their research report by saying, *"Bee pollen has regenerative properties for the body.* Bee pollen contains all the amino acids, mineral salts, vitamins, and enzymes in perfect proportion as needed by the organism."

As a further demonstration of bee pollen's powerful regenerating and rejuvenating effect, consider a paper coming out of Sarajevo, Yugoslavia. In a well-publicized study, Yugoslav researchers at the University of Sarajevo used oral bee pollen therapy on a group of impotent men. After a thirty day period, over half were documented as showing an increase in the production of sperm, probably because bee pollen's gonadatropic hormones act as a reproductive-gland stimulant.

AN OVERVIEW OF THE BENEFITS OF BEE POLLEN

There has been so much material published in just the past five years on bee pollen that it's difficult to bring you a full and complete condensation of the many, many benefits this super-rich and incredibly nutritious food offers.

AS A STOREHOUSE OF NUTRIENTS — Because the important part that the daily diet plays in keeping us well or making us sick has been well established, suffice it to say that any food which has been demonstrated to contain every element the body requires has to qualify as a super-food. Laboratory analysis of bee pollen confirms that it contains all the health-promoting live nutrients the body needs to sustain life itself.

What's more, bee pollen, the super-food, delivers these nutrients in perfectly balanced proportions. And, isn't it nice to know that Mother Nature has packaged it so superbly? You really don't have to take laboratory chemicals with your breakfast in order to get all the vitamins and minerals you need daily.

Dr. Alain Callais, Academie d'Agriculture, Paris, informs us that bee pollen is richer in essential protein than any animal source and says it contains more amino acids than beef, meat, eggs, or cheese of equal weight.

MEDICALLY SPEAKING

Centuries ago, Hippocrates said, "Let your food be your medicine; Let your medicine be your food." As a medicinal food, bee pollen scores high points again.

CANCER — As long ago as 1948, the Journal of the National Cancer Institute published results of a study conducted by Dr. William Robinson of the U.S.D.A. which determined that bee pollen contains an active anti-cancer element which has the power to slow the development of mammary tumors. Tumor growth increased in subjects in the control group not given bee pollen. Dr. Robinson concluded that bee pollen is a powerful cancer fighter and stated that "These experiments were based on the postulation that bee pollen contains an anti-carcinogenic principle which can be added to food."

Dr. Peter Hernuss, a practicing oncologist (cancer specialist) at the University of Vienna, reported a "noticeable decrease in the side-effects of radiation therapy" on women with uterine cancer when bee pollen was added to their diet. Hair loss, nausea and vomiting, loss of appetite, bladder and rectal inflammations, were greatly reduced in the women who took bee pollen during the course of their radiation therapy.

HEART HEALTH — A recent Polish study (May 1986) entitled "Effect of Pollen Extract on the Development of Experimental Atherosclerosis in Rabbits" conducted by a group of scientists at the Institute of Pharmacology & Toxicology, the Medical Academy (Szczecin, Poland) agrees with earlier research showing that the oral administration of pollen extract contributes significantly to the lowering of blood fat levels. In a group of lab animals fed a highly saturated fat diet, those protected by the addition of pollen extract were found to exhibit blood cholesterol levels reduced by 67 percent and liver cholesterol levels reduced by 45 percent.

The Polish scientists concluded that the oral administration of pollen extract significantly lowered serum lipid levels and modified lipid deposition in major arteries.

PROSTATE — A German/Swiss team of urologists reported that bee pollen ingestion proved most successful as a treatment of prostatitis and prevented the need for surgery in their study of over 170 men.

NATURAL ANTIBIOTIC — French scientists (Dr. Remy Chauvin, the Institute of Bee Culture, Paris, and Dr. E.

Lenormand, the Paris Child Preventatorium) report that bee pollen contains an extremely active natural antibiotic able to correct gastrointestinal tract functioning by destroying harmful bacteria.

British scientist Dr. G.J. Binding says, "Honeybee pollen provides an increased resistance to infection. It is a giant germ-killer in whose presence bacteria simply cannot exist."

THE BOTTOM LINE — In his popular book, *About Pollen,* author Carlson Wade sums it all up by saying, "The healing, rejuvenating and disease-fighting effects of this total nutrient are hard to believe, yet are fully documented. Aging, digestive upsets, prostate disease, sore throats, acne, fatigue, sexual problems, allergies, and a host of other problems have been successfully treated by the use of bee pollen."

THE ENDURANCE FOOD

WORLD-CLASS ATHLETES — Lasse Viren, the Finnish runner who took the gold in the 5000 and 10,000 meter events in both the 1972 and 1976 Olympic games says his speed and endurance come from bee pollen. The renowned Finnish coach, Antti Lananake, concurs. "Our studies," he says, "show bee pollen significantly improves the team's performance. Most of our athletes take a bee pollen food supplement.

Of all the running champions, the most famous is Steve Riddick, long called the "fastest man in the world." Riddick himself says, "After just two months on bee pollen, I felt as if my body shifted into a more powerful gear."

It took former U.S.S.R. Olympic track coach Remi Korchemny, now with the Pratt Institute in New York, to provide the answers. Korchemny mounted a two-year double-blind study with Pratt athletes, giving some bee pollen and some a placebo. His conclusions proved beyond doubt that bee pollen increased their crucial recovery time after stressed performance and enabled the athletes taking bee pollen to actually improve their performance the second time around.

Noel Johnson, the remarkable oldster who runs marathons at age 93 and who enjoys what he calls his "second lifetime" with the verve and zest of a young man, agrees. Johnson says,

"I'll be in better condition at 95 than I am today. I know now what you have to do to rebuild and keep your cells alive and I know what causes illness!"

FROM THE HIVE TO THE TABLE

How do we secure this potent rejuvenating and health-giving miracle food for ourselves? Bee pollen is harvested directly from the hive by means of a pollen-trap fitted with a smooth wire screen. In order to enter the hive, the worker bee must pass through the wire screen. It gently brushes off a portion of the pollen she has collected in her travels from flower to flower which then falls a few inches into a pollen drawer.

The beekeeper then periodically empties the drawer of its precious contents and *should* (some don't) refrigerate or freeze it to insure ultimate quality and freshness. When he has amassed a sufficient quantity, the beekeeper sells his bee pollen to one of several U.S. manufacturers for cleaning, processing, and packaging into product form.

CHOOSING THE RIGHT BEE POLLEN

We want to say a word here about quality bee pollens. If bee pollen is bee pollen, why not purchase the lowest priced product available? Well, my friends, while a rose by any other name may still smell as sweet, that premise does not apply when selecting a bee pollen source. There are good bee pollens that deliver a full measure of benefits and there are poor bee pollens. No matter what end product the manufacturer turns out, that product can only be as good as the bee pollen and other ingredients that went into its manufacture.

For instance, when you find bee pollen granules that are as hard as pebbles, you may be sure that they have been overdried at a heat high enough to destroy all the vital enzymatic action and reduce the nutrient value. You can easily apply this test yourself when purchasing bee pollen in granular form, but what about a capsulized or tableted product? It's very easy for a manufacturer to start with the cheapest grade Spanish pollen, for example. Once the product has been processed into capsules or tablets, there's just no way to determine what bee pollen has been used as its base ingredient.

Therefore, it's very important that you know and can trust the source of your bee pollen. By all means, shun all foreign products, some of which have been contaminated with carbon tetrachloride, most of which are heated, and all of which are old by the time they reach our shores.

In judging only the U.S. packagers of raw granules, there's more than one good brand available. Touted as being from the clean, sunwashed high mountains and deserts of the West, there are many good bee pollens available blended from different regions of the mid-West. They are not heat treated like some of the bee pollen imported from Spain or China, which are not recommended because of its questionable source. It is important that you always buy raw produced, unheated pollen, which are still enzyme-active. Any reputable health food outlet should have these in stock.

These companies supply a very high grade of blended bee pollens gathered exclusively in the clean mountains and high desert areas of the Western United States. Because no single-source pollen can supply a full complement of nutrients, a multi-source blend of bee pollens becomes obviously very important. In addition, these golden grains are harvested far from the environmental pollution that drifts over the cities, streets, and even the farms of the nation, assuring you of fresh, pure, uncontaminated bee pollen with all the goodness Mother Nature intended packed into each tiny granule. In fact, the virgin high deserts and mountains of the United States might just be some of the few places left in the world where man has not intruded with chemical fertilizers, insecticides, and other pollutants.

In addition, any excess moisture found in these harvests is removed with an exclusive cold process at around 70 degrees. Testing reveals that each golden grain delivered enzyme-active by these health food stores are of very good quality and guaranteed that they are produced without any harmful chemicals, and are still very potent. This is very important as an excellent source of nutrient-rich food which will give the body, if taken over a longer period of time, all the nutrients the human body needs for healthy functioning.

If you prefer the convenience of a premeasured dose, a powerful bee pollen product in an incredibly potent and unique new formulation is being sold under different trademarks, and is highly recommended. Each capsule contains top quality bee pollen, Siberian Ginseng, and the herb Gotu Kola, all integrated into a base of pure Royal Jelly. These additional ingredients both potentiate and synergistically increase the activity of the bee pollen, as well as providing important benefits of their own.

To show you exactly *why* we believe this excellent formulation is the best bee pollen combination product available, let's examine the active principles of each of the additional ingredients separately without regard to the bee pollen itself.

Royal Jelly — Royal jelly is called the 'rejuvenation factor,' and with very good reason. Science now recognizes the power of royal jelly to transform a single larvae (identical in every way to her sister larva) into the royalty of the hive, the Queen Bee. Just exactly how this mysterious nutrient accomplishes this miracle is still unknown, but it is a documented fact that the Queen Bee lives for up to *five years,* while the worker bees of the hive have a lifespan of mere weeks. The only difference between the two is that the Queen alone feasts on royal jelly for the whole of her extended lifespan.

Can royal jelly work this same miracle in man? Research coming out of the U.S.S.R. confirms that royal jelly contains *acetylcholine,* an important element shown to be lacking in the brains of Alzheimer's Disease victims on autopsy. The Soviet findings also state that royal jelly regulates blood pressure, stimulates the suprarenal glands, enhances the immune system, is effective in cases of arteriosclerosis and coronary deficiency, reduces cholesterol, and restores energy where it is lacking.

Siberian Ginseng — In contrast to the more common Korean ginseng (grown strictly for the lucrative commercial market in worn out fields), Siberian ginseng (*Eleutherococcus*) is expensive, but worth it. It is biologically active, very potent, and possesses all the properties that have made ginseng sought after for centuries.

In the traditional Chinese pharmacopeia of medicines, ginseng is known as the cure-all herb. It contains Vitamins A, B12, and E, plus thiamine, riboflavin, niacin, calcium, iron, phosphorus, potassium, magnesium, and sulphur. Ginseng is used in the Orient to overcome stress, to stimulate and improve brain function, as an antidote to drugs and toxins, to normalize blood pressure, reduce harmful cholesterol levels, and to energize and generally enhance health. Ginseng is considered a powerful youth restorer and is said to inhibit the aging process itself. As a preventive, this 'King of Herbs,' has no peer.

Gotu Kola — Gotu Kola (Hydrocotyle asiatica) is a natural herb that comes to us from the exotic islands of the Indian Ocean where the native doctors believe it contains remarkable stimulating and rejuvenating properties similar to those of ginseng (see above). An ancient Singhalese proverb says of Gotu Kola, "Eat two leaves a day to keep old age away." It contains Vitamins A, G, and K, and is rich in magnesium, plus small amounts of Vitamins E and B, and certain minerals. Herbologists use Gotu Kola as a blood purifier, to fight physical and mental fatigue, and as a senility preventive.

Note: All the bee pollen products mentioned in this chapter are available in major health food stores nationwide.

Chapter IX
An Introduction To The Macrobiotic Concept
The Yin & Yang Factors

In Oriental philosophy, the harmonious concept of *yin-yang* is depicted by a circle, with the light and dark half being equal. The yin-yang circle represents the universe and all that is in it.

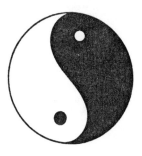

The Yin-Yang Symbol

YIN — Yin is conceived of as Earth, female, dark, passive, and absorbent. Yin is present in even numbers, valleys and waters, and is represented by the tiger, the color orange, and a broken line.

YANG — Yang is conceived of as Heaven, male, light, active, and penetrating. Yang is present in odd numbers, in mountains, and is represented by the dragon, the color blue, and an unbroken line.

The significance of the yin-yang circle permeates every aspect of Chinese thought and influences astrology, divination,

186

art, government, and even medicine. The human body, like matter in general, is made up of five elements: wood, fire, earth, metal, and water. Each of these elements is believed to be either yin or yang.

Controlling the proportions of yin and yang in the body is the basis of Chinese medicine. Chinese healers have used almost every conceivable natural substance therapeutically at one time or another to restore the balance of the yin and yang. The famous Chinese herbals from ancient times (over 1,000) were collected into one tremendous work, the *Pen-ts'ao kang-mu,* or Great Pharmacopoeia, by Li Shih-chen (1552-1578). This work totals 52 volumes and is still authoritative today.

Incidentally, a few of the better-known Chinese medicinals which have been adopted by Western civilization include: iron (anemia), castor oil (purge), kaolin (internal absorbent), aconite (an alkaloid pain reliever), camphor (relieves itching), chaulmoogra oil (leprosy), the herb *Mahuang,* which yields ephedrine (asthma) and the herb *Rauwolfia,* which yields reserpine (high blood pressure).

THE YIN-YANG THEORY

AN ANCIENT ORIENTAL PHILOSOPHY — In the body, oriental philosophy teaches that the two branches (ortho-sympathetic and para-sympathetic) of the nervous system are two halves of the same yin-yang circle. When all is well within the body, they work together in a complementary manner to control all the body's automatic functions. Illness and disease arise when the balance goes out of control. In the yin-yang theory, some sicknesses are caused by expansion (yin); some by contraction (yang).

For instance, a headache caused when the tissues and cells of the brain *contract* and press against each other is designated a *yang* sickness, while a headache caused by *expanding* tissues and cells pressing against each other is designated a *yin* sickness.

What happens because of an imbalance of the yin and yang factors can be seen very graphically when red blood cells are

187

altered by placing them in different solutions. Red blood cells placed in water (yin) absorb the water, expand, and finally burst. Red blood cells placed in a concentrated saline (salt) solution (yang), contract, shrink and shrivel. But, in a solution of 0.9% salt, the yin and yang are balanced and the cells remain virtually unchanged.

THE YIN-YANG CANCER THEORY

IS IT YIN OR YANG? — As the yin and yang concept relates specifically to cancer, consider the medical treatment of breast and prostrate malignancies. Female hormones (yin) can control prostate (yang) cancer. Male hormones (yang) can control breast cancer (yin). When the two halves of the yin-yang circle are harmoniously balanced, the malignancy is brought under control.

The macrobiotic diet is a completely natural means of changing the quality of the blood and cells and bringing them into a harmonious and healthy yin-yang balance.

THE MACROBIOTIC CONCEPT

EXTENDING LONGEVITY — We find that the dictionary defines *macrobiotics* as the art of lengthening the lifespan, especially by a vegetarian diet. Therefore, in the strictest sense of the word, anyone eating only plant foods grown in the region where he lives is following a macrobiotic diet.

However, we are examining here the precise macrobiotic concept as espoused, refined, and taught by Michio Kushi. It is based on the theory that all degenerative diseases, including cancer, are the result of a way of life that is out of harmony with the universal order of things.

For instance, an examination of the length of our digestive tract and the structure of our teeth certainly indicates that whole grains, vegetables, and beans — all of which require long chewing and a lengthy digestive process — were meant to be the principal foods of mankind, with certain variations appropriate to peoples living in vastly differing climates.

In the tropical regions of the world, the people traditionally eat a diet of locally-grown vegetables and fruits, while in the polar regions, the people subsist almost entirely on a diet of animal products native to their part of the world. For most of the peoples of the world who live in a temperate climate, the principal foods have always been whole grains and beans, along with local vegetables and fruits.

A DIETARY IMBALANCE — The disharmony, leading to a dietary imbalance which gives rise to disease, occurs when we deviate from the universal order as it was in the beginning and eat foods which were not ordained for our climatic range. According to the macrobiotic theory, it is these foods which upset the delicate harmonious yin-yang balance of the body and create disease when consumed over a period of time.

THE RELATIONSHIP BETWEEN DIET & DISEASE — Because new cells can only be manufactured from the elements provided in our diet, inferior cells are produced by an inferior diet. As a cellular dysfunction, the macrobiotic system shows that cancer is a prime example of improper food consumption over a long period of time.

When our food intake consists of high-quality nutrients, we get rid of any toxins through the normal elimination systems of the body via urination, bowel movements, respiration and perspiration. If our intake becomes excessive, the body shifts into another gear and employs additional and more violent elimination techniques, such as vomiting, diarrhea, frequent bowel movements and/or urination, sneezing, coughing, or a flash fever.

Whenever I suffered from a bout of flu as a child with the typical uncomfortable symptoms of diarrhea and vomiting, my mother always said, "That's the bad coming out of you, dear." It's true. The body automatically attempts to expel mucus, toxins, foreign matter, and harmful bacteria by all means at its command.

For instance, the macrobiotic concept explains that a chronic skin condition (or disease) may indicate that the eliminative systems of the body are over-loaded with toxins and the blood is no longer being properly cleansed. The sudden appearance of freckles and dark spots indicate the attempt of the body to discharge sugars and excessive carbohydrates, while white patches indicate the attempt of the body to get rid of excessive dairy products.

Further, when the bloodstream is clogged with fats and oils, the pores, sweat glands, and hair follicles may become completely blocked, resulting in chronic hard, dry skin. Dry skin is usually viewed as a lack of fats in the diet, but more often the reverse is true. When the blood is loaded with fats, moisture cannot reach the surface of the skin and dry, itchy skin results.

THE RELATIONSHIP BETWEEN ELIMINATION & DISEASE — When the eliminative systems of the body become exhausted or are prevented from efficient functioning by internal deposits of mucus or fat, the stage is set for serious illness. If these harmful toxins are not dissolved and discharged, they will be deposited in various parts of the body.

Typical sites of fat and mucus accumulations include the sinuses, the inner ear, the lungs, the breasts, the reproductive organs of both men and women, and the kidneys. Early symptoms created by these deposits may seem to be as far apart as a sinus headache is from a vaginal discharge or inflamed prostate, but actually they all result from the same cause: a buildup of toxic trash which the eliminative systems cannot remove.

If these toxins cannot be discharged, the body will continue storehousing the excess wherever it can. If high-quality nutrients are not immediately supplied to nourish cells and tissues, the cells will continue degenerating and a malignancy will flourish. Once the vital organs are infiltrated, survival hangs in the balance.

Think of what your kitchen would look like if for some reason you were unable to take out the garbage. You'd probably stuff all the trash and refuse in one corner and pile it up until the mess threatened to tip over. Then you'd be forced to select another site and another and another until your kitchen became so disgusting that you'd move out. Obviously, we can't vacate our bodies and move to a clean house. The only way we can clean up the mess we've made of our insides is by eating a proper diet. The macrobiotic diet is designed to clean up the mess.

HARMONY WITH NATURE — The macrobiotic concept also advocates both physical and mental exercise, a proven medical precept. Physical activity is necessary to stimulate circulation of the blood and lymph in order to eliminate the toxins present in the stagnant fluids of the body. Activities which stimulate body and mind assist in the production of energy and invigorate the digestive and nervous systems of the body as well.

Another important factor of the macrobiotic system is the distinction made between the *medically terminal* and the *macrobiotically treatable*. Certain medical procedures, such as intensive chemotherapy or radiation, result in a loss of some (or all) of the body's self-healing abilities. Macrobiotics teaches that the patient who has received drastic medical treatment must first recover from the toxic effects of that treatment before the macrobiotic diet can be effective against the malignancy.

THE CLEAN WAY TO EAT

PERSONALIZED NUTRITION — The standard macrobiotic diet is designed to provide the perfect balance of nutrients required for healthy cells. Only by encouraging the proliferation of healthy cells can we hope to guard against the development of any disease, including cancer. Macrobiotic foods assist the elimination systems of the body to dissolve and remove the toxins, fats, and mucus which can clog cells and tissues, leading to disease.

Macrobiotic experts caution that the same nutrient program is not right for everyone. If you are interested in pursuing the macrobiotic way of life, we urge you to contact the East West Foundation headquarters, whose address and phone number are provided at the close of this chapter. You will be guided to a highly qualified macrobiotic advisor in your area who will adjust the standard diet to fit your particular needs.

THE BASIC MACROBIOTIC DIET — The standard macrobiotic diet program is based on whole grains, beans, and cooked vegetables, along with certain supplementary foods, beverages and oriental condiments.

GRAINS — Whole cereal grains, including brown rice, whole wheat, oats, rye, corn, barley, buckwheat, and millet, should total between 50 and 60 percent of every meal.

VEGETABLES — Recommended vegetables include cabbage (green and Chinese), carrots, dandelion, burdock root, turnips (with tops), onions, squash (butternut and Hubbard), cauliflower, Swiss chard, bok choy, radish (daikon and regular types), watercress, and any other locally grown vegetables.

Total intake of the specific vegetables as recommended above should comprise between 25 and 30 percent of the day's nutrients. Up to one-third of the vegetables may be taken raw in a salad, but macrobiotic authorities say that persons with certain types of cancer should limit their intake of raw foods. Consult your qualified macrobiotic advisor to find out what's right for you.

Note: — Vegetables with a high acid or fat content, such as tomatoes, eggplant, potatoes, asparagus, spinach, sweet potatoes, beets, zucchini, yams, avocados, and green and red peppers, have no place in the macrobiotic diet.

BEANS & SEA VEGETABLES — A good health-food store or a shop offering Oriental specialties can supply the recommended mineral-rich sea vegetables, such as hiziki, kombu, wakame seaweed, nori, dulse, and Irish moss. The recommended low-fat beans include chickpeas, lentils, and azuki beans. Approximately 5 to 10 percent of the daily intake may include these delicacies, usually served as a side-dish or added to soups.

SOUPS — One or two small bowls of soup, seasoned with *miso* or *tamari* soy sauce, may be enjoyed daily. Prepare with the recommended beans, vegetables, and whole grains. Wakame seaweed should always be included.

BEVERAGES — Approved beverages include room-temperature spring water, any of the cereal grain coffees, roasted brown rice tea, roasted barley tea, dandelion tea, and roasted *kukicha* (bancha twig) tea.

192

SUPPLEMENTARY FOODS — A person in good health is allowed a small amount of low-fat *white fish,* plus a little fresh or dried *locally-grown fruit,* once or twice weekly. As a *snack,* roasted seeds, grains, or beans lightly seasoned with tamari, are permitted occasionally.

SEASONINGS — Sea salt, miso, tamari soy sauce, gomasio (sesame salt), kombu or wakame (seaweed) powders, Tekka, and Umeboshi plums are all delicious oriental condiments with specific benefits.

Note: — These seasonings are used sparingly. It is especially important to note that they are either *recommended* or *prohibited,* depending on the yin-yang balance of the ingestor, another reason why it's important to consult a qualified macrobiotic advisor before embarking on this type of diet.

MACROBIOTIC FOOD PREPARATION

BALANCED NUTRITION — There are several basic techniques in macrobiotic cooking that must be learned. In brief, a macrobiotic diet comprises healthy nutrient-rich foods containing a balanced complement of nutrients simply prepared. In the basic preparation, foods are steamed with a very little water. If oil is used, only moderate amounts of high-quality sesame or corn oil are allowed. Condiments add interesting flavor and certain condiments afford additional health benefits.

It is best to attend macrobiotic cooking classes. Classes may be available in your area. Take advantage of the opportunity to sample various dishes to find out what they are supposed to taste like and learn how to duplicate the specific culinary delights at home which will bring your body back into balance.

EATING CLEAN — If you are accustomed to sweet sugary foods, greasy fatty foods, heavy protein foods, excessively spiced and salted foods, and/or the thrice daily consumption of dairy products, prepare for an adventure. Be aware that your over-stimulated taste buds have become dulled and clogged, along with the rest of your body.

You will probably find the clean macrobiotic diet bland and perhaps even tasteless in the beginning. If you are one of those misguided individuals who is actually proud to say, "I live to eat," and who stubbornly persists in overindulging in spite of the consequences, it's time to change your style.

The following pages outline a few inspiring and documented case histories of those who have embraced macrobiotics. These stories show very clearly the health benefits that the clean way to eat and live has brought into their lives.

Once you have made the decision to *"eat to live,"* contact the East West Foundation headquarters for the name and address of a branch in your area. All Foundation affiliates offer counseling services, cooking classes, and courses in the macrobiotic philosophy.

The East West Foundation
17 Station Street
Brookline, MA 02146
Phone: 413-623-5741

The case histories that follow are adapted from material which first appeared in the *East West Journal*, address given above. (All rights reserved.) We extend special thanks to the *East West Journal* for permitting us to present this exceptionally strong empirical evidence of the undeniable power of the macrobiotic way of life.

DOCUMENTED MEDICAL EVIDENCE

MACROBIOTICS vs PROSTATE CANCER — In 1975, a gentleman in his mid-fifties, Mr. I.M., was diagnosed as suffering from prostate cancer and began conventional medical treatment. The disease spread into his spine, his right hip, and his right shoulder. Medical treatment included surgery in which a portion of one testicle was removed (a partial *orchiectomy*), radiation therapy, and chemotherapy. Mr. M. also took hormones orally. He was in continual pain and vomited violently for 12 hours after every round of chemotherapy. Understandably, he became very weak and feeble. In spite of these measures, Mr. M.'s health continued to deteriorate.

Near the end of 1980, Mr. M. absolutely refused further chemotherapy, but agreed to continue with the oral hormones. He consulted an M.D. who recommended macrobiotics and got him started correctly on the macrobiotic lifestyle. Almost immediately, his appetite improved and his energy began to come back. Just one month after beginning the macrobiotic diet, Mr. M. decided on his own to cut his hormone intake in half. Within six months, he was no longer in pain and felt so invigorated that he stopped taking the hormones entirely.

Mr. M. attributed his dramatic improvement entirely to macrobiotics. He decided to have a bone scan to confirm his feeling that the cancer was being conquered. Radiologists reading his x-rays found that there was an obvious shrinking and clearing evident in all previous sites of the malignancy. Expert oncologists had to agree that the hormone therapy alone could not have accounted for the reversal of the disease evident in Mr. M.'s diagnostic bone scan.

Mr. M. says, "I follow the macrobiotic way of life. I am totally convinced that we are what we eat and that we literally destroy our bodies with the poor quality of foods we consume. At age 60, I continue to work full time and also often spend evening hours doing work. I maintain a reasonable amount of exercise and look upon cancer as something we can overcome with diet and determination. Our amazing bodies can heal themselves if we furnish them with the proper nourishment and eliminate that which is harmful."

MACROBIOTICS vs CERVICAL CANCER — At the age of 27, Miss D.G., a Licensed Practical Nurse, was diagnosed as having cancer of the cervix. After several Pap smears and two biopsies, she was treated by a surgical procedure known as *conization* in which several layers of tissue were scraped away from all around the cervix. Unfortunately the cancer cells reappeared.

Because her doctor recommended she continue taking birth control pills, Miss G. decided to change doctors. As an LPN, Miss G. knew hormones could stimulate the growth of a malignancy. Her next doctor was more conservative and agreed to monitor her condition closely by taking Pap smears every three months. The smears continued to read positive.

On her own, Miss G. began making certain changes in her diet, eating less in general and reducing her intake of fats, refined foods, and chemically processed foods drastically. It was not until about a year later that she was introduced to macrobiotics. She embraced the macrobiotic regimen completely and discovered the principle of balance as emphasized in macrobiotic teachings.

After just six months on macrobiotics, Miss. G.'s Pap smears read negative. Her doctor termed it a "spontaneous remission," but she knew better. Miss G. says, "The only thing I changed was my diet! The conization hadn't worked. The cancer cells had appeared again after that had been done. Now, after 12 years, there has still been no sign of the cancer cells reappearing." The additional benefits Miss G. has experienced on the macrobiotic regimen are truly amazing. In addition to curing her cervical cancer, her hypoglycemia has disappeared; she no longer suffers monthly with PMS; the chronic lower back pain she experienced periodically no longer troubles her; the stuffed-up nose and blocked sinuses which had been with her since she was a child have cleared; her hemorrhoids disappeared; a psoriasis-type condition she suffered on her scalp and the acne pustules which were always with her are gone forever; she has lost a tendency to put on weight and reports her body has become more soft, feminine and graceful.

Miss G. says, "I would like to see nurses learn more about teaching patients what they can do for themselves, particularly in the area of macrobiotic, natural treatments. I think that nutrition and the link between diet and disease should become an integral part of nursing training. My own experience has shown me that this is just one more of the many wonderful things macrobiotics has to offer us today."

MACROBIOTICS vs OVARIAN CANCER — The doctors diagnosed chronic *endometriosis* (an infection of the lining of the uterus) and told Miss. T.G. that she would never be able to have children. Before she was twenty, Miss. G. underwent an operation to remove one ovary and a Fallopian tube. She was put on oral hormone therapy, causing her to lose all her hair.

Miss G. moved to another city and continued to suffer intermittent pain, which increased to the point that she went to a gynecologist. He determined that her endometriosis had flared up and also found a cyst the size of a small tennis ball. He recommended a complete hysterectomy, but Miss G. rebelled and moved into a macrobiotic study house. After just three months of clean macrobiotic eating, the cyst disappeared.

The attractive young woman's future husband took her to meet with Michio Kushi, the President of the East West Foundation. Miss G. says, "Michio could tell simply by looking at me that my left ovary had been removed and the remaining one was still very diseased. He also said I had a tumor growing in my descending colon and that I had jaundice. I was very inspired and convinced to follow the diet he recommended.

"For the next year, I ate very simply. Mentally, I was much improved. I became very meticulous about macrobiotics. Anytime I cheated, I would feel severe internal pain. As long as I continued with external treatments and the recommended diet, the pain would be nonexistent. One day I discharged a lump of cancerous tissue with my bowel movement. I began to feel much lighter as my intestines also improved."

Within a year, Miss G. married and the couple decided to have a baby. The pregnancy was easy and comfortable, as was the birth of a healthy son. Her second child followed a few years later with no complications, despite the prognosis of the medical doctors who had told her she would never be able to have children.

The happy young mother now says, "I know I was very arrogant and very sick. I had thought that macrobiotics would take the fun out of my life, but my life is much simpler and much more fulfilling than ever before. It's my sincere hope that many, many people will come to the macrobiotic way of life whether they are sick or not."

MACROBIOTICS vs WIDESPREAD CANCER — "You have a two percent chance of living out the year," the physicians bluntly told then 23 year old J.J. and his fiance, I.K. The cancer which had begun as a pea-sized lump on J.J.'s left testicle had spread into both lungs, his left kidney, and his neck.

After the complete surgical removal of his left testicle, J.J. was barely allowed time for his body to recover from the trauma of surgery before the prescribed chemotherapy treatments began. The routine was seven days of continuous treatment in the hospital, after which he was sent home to recoup and recover. When his blood count returned to normal, within two or three weeks, he had to return to the hospital for another bout of drugs.

J.J. suffered the typical side-effects of the chemotherapy, vomiting violently and spasmodically, and became weaker and more and more feeble. His condition was monitored constantly to determine the effects of the chemotherapy treatments, but the results were not encouraging. After the third series of treatments, the doctors recommended an experimental drug (*sis platinum*) be used in conjunction with the chemical treatments. After intravenous administration of the new drug, J.J. went into violent, racking convulsions. Of the experience, he says, "I felt as if I could just let go and die right there."

That night, he dreamed his mother (deceased) came to him and told him, "Go to St. Joseph's." St. Joseph's Oratory in Montreal, Canada is the home of Brother Andre, renowned for his healing miracles. Pilgrims to St. Joseph's travel the multitude of steps leading to the cathedral on the top of the mountain on their knees to show their humility and reverence. The dream made a powerful impression on J.J. and he felt compelled to go up St. Joseph's steps on his knees to pray for help.

When he was sent home from the hospital to recuperate, J.J. and his fiance discovered her mother was practicing macrobiotics for a lupus condition. This was their first introduction to this way of life. They purchased books and contacted their local East West Foundation for more information. Upon visiting the Foundation, J.J. was told of the diet he should follow.

The young couple felt the first stirrings of a faint hope, but it was time for J.J. to return to the hospital for another round of chemotherapy and sis platinum. Afterwards, the battery of tests showed that the tumors in his lungs were still present and the tumor in his neck had not changed. Although his blood tests had improved, the fact that the tumors were still present after such intense treatment was not considered a good sign.

J.J.'s teeth were extremely loose, his hair was gone, the membranes inside his mouth were encrusted with sores, he couldn't stop vomiting, and was barely able to walk across the room. It appeared to his loving fiancee that the treatment was worse than the disease and she finally asked him, "What do you want to die of, my love?" Together, they decided to begin macrobiotics. J.J. stopped all medical treatment, including chemotherapy, and never resumed it. He left the hospital determined to make a pilgrimage to St. Joseph's. His fiancee accompanied him.

As J.J. made the tortuous climb up the mountain steps on his knees, he prayed at each step for his relatives, ancestors, and friends who needed help, but not for himself. J.J. grew up with the strong belief that God knows what you need; you don't have to ask. With each step up, he experienced a warm feeling that he would practice macrobiotics, the tumors would disappear, and he would regain his health.

And so it happened.When the young couple returned home, they began studying macrobiotics and put the program into practice. Once he began the macrobiotic diet, J.J.'s strength returned quickly. After a year, blood tests showed no signs of cancer and the tumor in his neck had virtually disappeared. His wasted body was fleshed out with healthy muscle, his hair had grown back, and he was once again trim and fit. A very vital young man, J.J. himself says he feels better now than when he was playing high school football.

In J.J.'s case, a great number of factors came together to bring him back from the edge of the grave itself. He had the unswerving love of a very determined young woman who refused to give up; he had the good fortune to discover macrobiotics and the good sense to put into practice the macrobiotic program which restored his inner balance; and, perhaps most important of all, he had a deep and abiding faith in a powerful, loving God and a rare belief in miracles.

Chapter X

Visualization Therapy

Conquering Disease Through Positive Imagery

A DREAM OF PAST & FUTURE WONDERS — It is said that an ancient super-race once (or perhaps more than once) existed on Earth and will come yet again. Faint representations of what we like to believe were incredible beings still remain, now eroded, but deeply cut in cliff walls or chiseled into stone figures or painted on faded and chipped frescoes. If the old legends are to be believed, these humanoid creatures either descended from Mount Olympus or escaped from a cooling and dying star in the chariots of the gods, but (in our innermost hearts) we cling to the belief that there once existed an advanced and mystical people who were somehow privy to all the secrets of the universe.

These wondrous beings were forever young. The women were all meltingly beautiful and the men were all stalwart and handsome. Illness and disease and wars and financial hardship and every-day problems with the children (or the boss or a spouse) simply didn't exist for these fortunate creatures. They could not conceive of such horrors afflicting 'the immortals' (as they thought of themselves) and allowed these mundane concerns to be visited upon those of us who are mortals instead. And, guess what? We have meekly accepted all these horrors and taken them upon ourselves.

Let us assume for a moment that the ancient legends are true. That a mighty and invincible people, far more advanced than ourselves, once did walk among us on planet earth. What would it have been that set them so far above us? If we reject the idea that all-powerful gods and goddesses mysteriously endowed with mystical powers from on-high occasionally deign to visit us, and instead consider the possibility that humanoid creatures from another star system far ahead of us in knowledge just might have reached earth in the misty recesses of our collective past, the one thing that would have given them the edge is *mind power.*

THE GHOST IN THE MACHINE

THE BRAIN — The brain is a mass of gray nerve tissue protected from harm by the bony cage of the skull. It is the brain which regulates and coordinates the voluntary and involuntary systems of the entire body. Tiny electrical motor impulses work through the nervous system to transmit the appropriate message to specific glands and muscles to initiate a variety of activities. Blood circulation and breathing are regulated automatically through the cardiac, vasomotor, and respiratory reflex centers.

Medical science says the mind is: "An integration of the functions of the brain resulting in the ability to perceive surroundings, to have emotions, imagination, memory, and will, and to process information in an intelligent manner." (Taber's Cyclopedic Medical Dictionary) This is as good a working definition as any, but science still cannot open the skull, dissect the brain, and point to 'the mind.'

THE MIND — If we look upon the body as a machine, and the brain (and central nervous system) as the computer which programs and runs the machine, we still haven't recognized *the mind,* and it is the mind that makes the whole system work. Before the teachings of Sigmund Freud gained wide acceptance, most of us would have agreed that the idea of subconscious mental phenomena was impossible. But, since Freud opened the door, the power of the mind to affect the body has been demonstrated time and time again.

201

Since the dawn of time, mankind has attempted to define and put a label on the mind. In *The Concept of Mind,* (Barnes & Noble, NY) Gilbert Ryle called it: "The dogma of the Ghost in the Machine." Ryle says, "Minds are not in space, nor are their operations subject to mechanical laws. The workings of one's mind are not witnessable by other observers; its career is private."

It is a documented fact that a large portion (up to 90 percent) of the brain remains unused. This vast untapped power can be harnessed and put to work to accomplish many wonders. Stroke victims, with therapy, can often train their brains to use new pathways for speech and motor functions when the old ones have been destroyed. If a physician finds it possible to excise (cut out) a cancerous brain tumor and, in the doing, severs important sensory nerves, another portion of the brain may be able to take over. Considering these facts, it really shouldn't be surprising to learn that we can harness some of our unused *mind power* and use it to heal the body of cancer and other terrible diseases as well.

PROCEED WITH CAUTION — Although it is true that the mind possesses powers science can't explain, it would be unwise in the extreme to rely solely on the following visualization techniques and either put off seeing a qualified doctor or arbitrarily decide to discontinue medical treatment if you are under the care of a physician for any condition, especially cancer.

VISUALIZATION THERAPY

THE SIMONTON APPROACH — Dr. O. Carl Simonton (Cancer Counseling & Research Center, Dallas, Texas) explains that cancer, in particular, will flourish in a body whose owner is in a state of deep despair. Dr. Simonton says that psychological forces in the innermost recesses of the mind can actually assist the growth and development of a malignancy. On the other hand, Dr. Simonton teaches that psychological mind power can be consciously activated to battle and conquer disease.

After psychological testing and an intensive physical examination, Dr. Simonton puts his patients into psychotherapy.

During these sessions, he teaches his patients the technique of what he calls *imaging*. His patients learn to stimulate their immune-defense system by imagining a fierce internal battle proceeding in the area of their cancers, with the healthy cells conquering the malignant cells.

Dr. Simonton makes it clear that he has completely rejected orthodox medical treatment, including chemotherapy and radiation. Dr. Simonton healed himself of skin cancer on his nose over a period of one year. Although we have no case histories available, he cites statistics showing that patients under his care who practice his technique of imaging have up to twice the life expectancy that might be expected for their particular forms of cancer.

THE SALOV APPROACH — Leslie H. Salov, M.D. (Director of the Vision & Health Center, Whitewater, Wisconsin) is a very effective teacher of visualization therapy. He reports notable success with a toddler of four and one-half years afflicted with five *angiomas* (blood tumors) behind her left eyeball. (Children are particularly good candidates for visualization therapy because their minds are not cluttered with negatives.)

Just three days after little Sara's left eye first became red and swollen, the tumors had progressed to the point where her eyeball was forced out of its socket almost three-quarters of an inch. Sara's eyesight was deteriorating rapidly in that eye and medication prescribed by her ophthalmologist had to be discontinued because small hemorrhages in the eye occurred. It was apparent that the condition was extremely serious and Sara's parents were told that the eyeball would have to be removed along with the tumors. The rapidly growing tumors were constricting the optic nerve itself and stressing vital blood vessels.

When they learned of Dr. Salov's program, Sara's parents took her to him immediately. The doctor sat the child on his knee and explained to her, very gently, in plain language exactly what her problem was, how the tumors were growing, and what would happen. He showed her pictures and took much time with the toddler to make sure she understood her condition. **Dr. Salov** asked Sara to think about what was happening to her and then draw him a picture. The little girl said shyly that she would do that.

The following day, Sara's parents brought her back to Dr. Salov and she gave him the crayoned picture she had drawn. The picture showed an eye with the tumors behind it. The eye had an angry face, but with her mother's help, Sara had printed 'I love you' and written her name below the phrase. Dr. Salov was very pleased with her childish but clear understanding of her condition.

The next step was to teach Sara his technique of what he calls *visual imagery.* Dr. Salov told Sara that her mother would give her a bucket and a small syringe filled with red water. Sara was instructed to look at the picture she had crayoned of her eye with the five tumors glaring out from behind it. As she squeezed the red water in spurts out of the syringe into the bucket, she was to imagine that the tumors were in the red water. As she squeezed, the bulb would become smaller and smaller as the water spurted out. Sara was told that the tumors behind her eye would also become smaller and smaller until they disappeared.

After just one month, Sara's protruding left eye had begun to resettle into its socket, showing that the tumors were being absorbed into her system. With continued visual imagery, by eleven months later, Sara's vision was almost normal and her pretty little face had lost its deformed look. She is now completely cured.

Dr. Salov developed his particular visual imagery technique when he himself found he was losing his eyesight due to a severe degenerative condition. After being forced to retire from practice because of failing vision, Dr. Salov heard of visualization therapy and began practicing it on himself at home. At first skeptical at what he thought of as totally outside the realm of science, he became convinced and a strong advocate of this type of treatment when he successfully restored seventy-five percent of his visual acuity.

THE RUDEMAN APPROACH — A Californian by the name of Sheldon Rudeman successfully healed himself of lung cancer. When his physician told him he had less than two years to live, Rudeman decided to prove the doctor wrong. He began an intensive program of visualization therapy on himself and, cured of the lung cancer that orthodox medicine said was his death sentence, became a visualization counsellor himself six years later — a full four healthy years after he was supposed to die of the disease.

Rudeman tells of a seven-year old boy suffering with advanced renal (kidney) cancer. He taught young Michael how to visualize the cancer as a monster invading his body and trying to destroy him. Mike drew pictures of the cancer monster and showed the forces of good attacking it. Rudeman asked Michael just how long it would take for the forces of good to conquer the cancer monster. Michael said the monster would be gone by the time he was eight years old, six months away.

In an interview when he was a normal active eleven year old boy and in what his doctor termed "full remission," Michael was asked how he destroyed the cancer monster. He said, "I just shot it up with glue!"

THE POWER OF POSITIVE IMAGERY

UNDERSTANDING THE SUBCONSCIOUS — Dr. Jonas Miller (Sarasota, Florida) says it is very important to be truthful with your subconscious. Dr. Miller tells the true story of a physician acquaintance to illustrate this point. This physician, the victim of a serious heart condition, made a tape recording saying "Every day in every way my heart is getting stronger and stronger." Every night he put the tape recorder under his pillow where these words were fed into his subconscious over and over while he slept. But one morning the doctor was found dead in his bed of a heart attack with the tape recorder still repeating its hopeful message time and time again.

Dr. Miller explains: "Never lie to your subconscious. Don't say you're well when you're sick. Don't say you're getting better when you're not, as the doctor was doing. He was not acknowledging his sickness and was trying to cover over a truth, but his subconscious knew better. If you make a statement which is untrue, your subconscious will know you're lying and won't follow through with the desired results."

According to Dr. Miller, who is also an ordained minister, the correct way to prepare your subconscious is to first recognize your illness, reject it, and then feed it a complete picture of robust good health. A woman with a cancerous growth on her face once came to Dr. Miller saying, "I've got this cancer and I need prayer." He instructed her to stop identifying with the malignancy and claiming it as her own, which she did by saying *"I've got this cancer,"* and instead to credit it to the devil. With perfect faith, the woman did as Dr. Miller instructed and the growth disappeared.

HOW TO PRACTICE VISUALIZATION THERAPY

GETTING STARTED ON YOUR OWN — If you are unable to find a doctor or counselor to prepare a scenario encompassing visualization techniques for you, you can develop your own. First, acknowledge your disease, but let your subconscious know that it is an unwelcome invader which should be eliminated. Imagine the 'good guys (the lymphocytes and macrophage cells of your immune system) attacking and defeating the 'bad guys' (the diseased or cancerous cells).

You might picture a white knight in shining armor hacking away at dragon tentacles, or a David aiming his slingshot unerringly at an ugly Goliath, or a faceless monster being vanquished by purity. First develop a mental image of your disease to give it reality and sketch it to reinforce your subconscious concept. Then picture the very epitome of good in any guise you may imagine and draw in the good image attacking the evil image. Don't worry if your artistic ability is zero. Whether you're using stick people or geometric shapes or what appears to be a mish-mash really doesn't matter. The idea of putting the images on paper is to impress your subconscious with the process it will then initiate in your body.

If you wish to add props, such as Sara's syringe of red water, to further reinforce and impress your subconscious, go ahead. In fact, if your imagination is a little rusty and you are having difficulty visualizing the healing process in the way you want it to proceed, adding props is a very good idea.

You might want to start with a very large 'monster' potato, for instance, and cut away many small slivers every day while visualizing an internal tumor being gradually reduced by a magic knife of pure gold. Because visualization therapy is not by any means an instantaneous cure, once the original potato has become smaller, start in on another of medium-size and continue the slicing away process day by day to reinforce your mental image of a tumor disappearing sliver by sliver.

Or you might want to do a series of daily drawings showing a huge mass of diseased cells being consumed bit by tiny bit day by day by a simple sunshine yellow pac-man cartoon shape. Your daily sketches should show the mass continually becoming less and less as you visualize the yellow pac-man gobbling away at the diseased mass within your body.

On the other hand, you might opt to relax in some quiet place and concentrate on running mental images through your mind depicting the conquering hero vanquishing the dread enemy. Simply directing your immune system to marshall its forces of lymphocytes and macrophages and sending them on a search and destroy mission is equally effective without any outside props as long as your visual images are strong, purposeful, and powerful.

TWO DAILY SESSIONS — Most authorities recommend practicing visualization for at least two twenty minute periods every day. During this time, you are directed to concentrate intensely on developing and sustaining mental images of your disease being gradually conquered and eliminated by strong forces of good. Once your mental images are strong, your subconscious will deliver these images to you at will. At odd times during the day, call up the images to reinforce the immune system and give it a boost. It's also a good idea to begin and close the day with a few additional minutes of powerful visualization so that your subconscious is continually kept aware of its role.

HOW LONG WILL IT TAKE? — Who knows? The success of visualization therapy is dependent on many factors, including the strength of your commitment and your ability to persuade your subconscious to direct the internal forces of the body to attack and conquer. It is not a recognized and universally accepted medical or scientific procedure, but a great many documented cures have been accomplished by this means. *Visualization therapy does work.* — If you decide to use this dynamic technique to eliminate disease and restore health in your life, let us know of your experiences. We care.

In closing, I'd like you to meet the young lady, Sara, mentioned in this chapter, who vividly illustrates the effectiveness of visualization therapy.

A special X-ray exam of the girl's skull revealed the cause of the protruding eye - five blood tumors, called lymphangiomas, had grown behind Sara's eyeball. They were pressing on veins and the optic nerve. The doctors said if the pressure was not relieved, the optic nerve could die. Sara would lose the vision in her eye. A decompression surgery followed, but Sara's eyesight had already deteriorated drastically.

Sara's parents were told nothing more could be done until the eyeball was completely exposed from its socket. Then, doctors would surgically remove the eyeball, tumors and glands inside her left eye socket. In time, an artificial eye could be implanted.

"We first saw Sara in November," Salov said. "Before the end of December, the absorption of the tumors from behind the eye, as well as the restoration and positioning of the eye to its normal orbital depth, demonstrated more than my description of words, the phenomenal, awesome power of the mind... and the too often latent, unappreciated ability to heal ourselves, which is God-given."

A year later, Sara's vision was almost normal. There were no scars or disfigurements - just the twinkling eyes of a happy child.

A Family's Faith, A Little Girl's Courage, And Wholistic Ophthalmology Combine to Save An Eye That Was All But Lost.

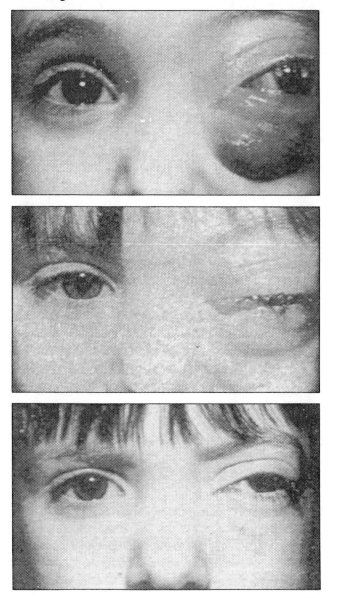

continued, next page

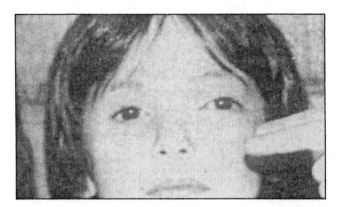

These photos, as painfully graphic as they are, illustrate the dramatic reversal of Sara's eye condition. We chose not to use those taken at the height of her condition, as they could prove embarrassing to her and repulsive to some readers. Even so, these illustrations aptly show the remarkable recovery experienced by this youngster and her fertile imagination.

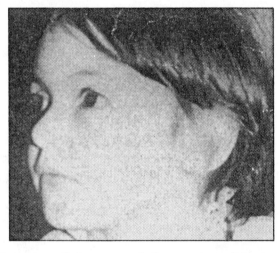

Those interested in more information on visualization therapy may contact Leslie H. Salov, MD at the Vision and Health Center, W 3064 Piper Road, Whitewater, WI 53190, phone 414-473-7361. The doctor asks that you include a business-sized, stamped, self-addressed envelope for replies.

Chapter XI
Little-Known Cancer Preventatives & Some Avoidable Carcinogens

Controversial Findings From Around The World

In 1962, 170 persons in every 100,000 died of cancer. In 1982, the tally was 185 persons in every 100,000. On the surface, it appears that the incidence of cancer has gone up an alarming 9 percent in the last twenty years. But the American Cancer Society points out that it is the escalation of lung cancer rates (tied inescapably to a proportionate escalation in smoking) which has caused the increase. The ACS points out that the death rate for most other cancers remains approximately the same as it was in 1962. According to ACS projections, over one million Americans will be diagnosed as having some form of cancer in 1986.

Is that good enough? Dr. John C. Bailar doesn't think we've received sufficient value for our money. The well respected *New England Journal of Medicine* (May 1986) carried an article authored by Dr. John C. Bailar of the School of Public Health at Harvard. Dr. Bailar contends that we are losing the war against cancer and puts forth a recommendation that he believes will go a long way toward solving the problem. Dr. Bailar suggests that researchers concentrate instead on discovering ways to prevent the disease from occurring in the first place. He suggests that for every dollar spent on researching a cure, two dollars be spent on researching preventive measures. We agree. A preventive approach will certainly benefit all of us now living and may eliminate the spectre of cancer hanging heavy over the heads of future generations as well.

Researchers around the world have been coming up with some startling data. Although most of the findings from various parts of the globe regarding cancer preventives and/or cancer therapies are based on sound scientific theory and are founded on impressive clinical research, very little of this vital information has been made available to the American public until now.

LAETRILE—A CASE IN POINT

The name *Laetrile,* an apricot pit formula which was developed at the John Beard Memorial Foundation in San Francisco, is a registered trademark coined in 1952 by its discoverer, Ernst Krebs, Jr. Laetrile is a combination of the term *laevorotary* (having the ability to turn polarized light to the left) and *nitrile* (an organic compound in which nitrogen exists with all three of the displaced hydrogen atoms). Laetrile is commonly misused as a generic term for *amygdalin* (B-17).

AMYGDALIN — Amygdalin is found in over a thousand foods, one or more of which most of us eat every day. Lettuce, corn, kidney beans, sugar cane, millet, cassava, sorghum, lima beans, sweet potatoes and linseed all contain amygdalin. Strawberries, raspberries, blackberries, boysenberries, cranberries, elderberries, mulberries, gooseberries, huckleberries, loganberries and chokeberries furnish amygdalin. (Note: Amygdalin is more abundant in wild berries than in cultivated.) And, although we don't usually crunch the hard pits of the following popular fruits, amygdalin is also present in the seeds of apples, apricots, bitter almonds, cherries, peaches, plums, and prunes. (Note: Sweet almonds contain very little amygdalin.)

Amygdalin contains a natural cyanide compound which is not toxic in the human body and this natural form of cyanide is of immense value in cancer treatment. The malignant cell contains a special enzyme which releases the poison in amygdalin. The poison, in turn, attacks the malignant cell and assists in its destruction. Normal cells do not contain this special enzyme, do not release the cyanide, and therefore remain unchanged and unharmed.

When a correlation of data provides a comparison of people who ingest foods high in amygdalin versus those who do not, we may find an important clue to why some individuals contract cancer while others do not. If we are continually providing our body with foods containing amygdalin, known to attack and destroy cancer cells, how then can a malignancy grow and spread? Amygdalin will almost certainly prove to be an exceptionally efficient cancer-preventive.

The difference between amygdalin and Laetrile is that Laetrile contains amygdalin changed by a patented process from a glucoside to glucuronic acid. When amygdalin itself is ingested, either in foods or as an extracted compound, the conversion process from glucose to glucuronic acid takes place in the liver. Because Laetrile is already a glucuronic acid, the body does not have to initiate the conversion process. (Note: Extracted amygdalin is highly unstable in liquid form. Only dry, crystallized amygdalin is considered therapeutically active.)

Even though bitter almonds, probably the most abundant source of natural amygdalin, have been used in Chinese herbal medicine since 2800 B.C., the U.S. Food & Drug Administration does not consider the natural compound Laetrile a food, but has instead termed it a "drug." As the champion and sponsor of Laetrile, the McNaughton Foundation has handled all the red-tape and paper work necessary to bring this compound to the world.

After Phase I testing was completed by the FDA, Laetrile was pronounced nontoxic. By the end of 1978, more than 20 states had ruled that their citizens had a right to choose Laetrile as a holistic and nontoxic treatment for cancer and all seemed well. But approximately a year later, the National Cancer Institute filed an I.N.D. (Investigational New Drug) application and Phase II testing of Laetrile was scheduled. Phase II testing is allowed *only* after Phase I testing proves that the material being tested is not toxic in prescribed amounts. However, at a meeting of the Society of Clinical Oncology on April 30, 1981, Charles Moertel, M.D., of the prestigious Mayo Clinic announced, "Laetrile has been tested. It is not effective." Laetrile advocates believe that the Mayo Clinic test was faulty, but the bottom line is that this form of amygdalin is no longer legal in the U.S.

DATELINE EUROPE

Although the nutritional approach to treatment and prevention of cancer and the other degenerative diseases is rapidly gaining support in the U.S., our cousins across the ocean seem to be a step ahead of us.

GERMANY — One of the most comprehensive treatises on disease prevention and cure currently in publication is a scholarly work by the world-famous Hans Nieper, M.D. entitled *Revolution in Technology, Medicine, & Society.* Although this important book has been published in English as well as German, you won't find it in many local bookstores or even your neighborhood library. This work delves deeply into the causes of all the common diseases of civilization, including cancer, and explains some of the most successful methods of both treatment and prevention.

GENE-REPAIRING TREATMENT — Dr. Nieper says, "Some of the gene-repairing therapeutic measures for cancer, as well as protective measures for cancer, are already available and others will be added. Therapy should be applied immediately after the first discovery of, or operation on, a malignant tumor. This is mandatory. Any waiting game is fundamentally wrong. Modern gene-repairing therapy is practically nontoxic. It represents, so to speak, an imitation of the cancer defenses of the body. Today there is no longer any doubt about its high clinical value." In this chapter, we will briefly detail the findings, preventives, and treatments discussed in this serious work, plus outline the factors which are known to add to the risk of contracting cancer.

DIETARY CONSIDERATIONS

THE FOOD FACTOR - As a very graphic example of the chemical changes certain foods exert within the body, consider the case of a respected German physician which was presented at the Baden-Baden cancer congress. This physician used himself as an experimental tool to prove a point. After eating a meal of fried chicken, the doctor demonstrated that the malignant tumor in his neck was well-nourished and grew rapidly. In direct contrast, he found that a whole grain diet of millet caused the tumor to be drastically reduced. In fact, the millet diet proved more effective in shrinking the tumor than orthodox chemotherapy.

This case alone proves that the body is influenced daily by nutrient intake. Diet plays a vital part in the *day-to-day* functioning of the body and does not merely affect the body over the long-term, as most authorities believe.

According to Dr. Nieper, the dietary recommendations of the U.S. Department of Health, Education & Welfare for a cancer-protective diet are incomplete in that there is no mention of the importance of Vitamins C and D2, magnesium, molybdenum, selenium, and beta-carotene in reducing the risk of contracting cancer.

OBESITY — Another factor which is stressed by knowledgeable oncologists is the importance of *under-eating*. Unfortunately, Americans are particularly fond of overeating. While an occasional holiday feast will not increase the long-term risk of developing cancer (as long as only the proper foods are enjoyed), carrying even a mere ten pounds over your ideal weight can add to your risk. A U.S. study conducted by Bayer Pharmaceuticals clearly showed that the incidence of cancer

213

was reduced in laboratory mice especially bred to develop mammary cancer when they were consistently underfed. The healthiest exercise in the world still remains pushing yourself away from the table after a meager meal. Clearly, gluttony is one of the deadliest of the seven deadly sins.

Although German health authorities have not publicized a cancer-preventive diet, the recommendations contained in Dr. Nieper's book, *Revolution in Technology, Medicine, & Society,* follow. It is interesting to note that these recommendations are very similar to the recommendations of the U.S. National Research Council.

PREFERRED FOODS
- Whole grains (favored grains are oatmeal and millet)
- Skim Milk
- Fish (in limited quantity)
- Fruit and Fiber-Rich Vegetables (cooked and raw)
- Carrot Juice (freshly prepared)
- Pancreatic Enzyme Supplements
- *Omniflora** capsules and *Eupalan** bifidum flora containing milk
  (* German preparations)

RESTRICTED FOODS
- No Meat; No Sausage (6 or 7 ounces meat per week is permitted in cases of exhaustion, lack of blood protein, or cachexia)
- Little Cheese
- Very Little Sugar
- Very Little Fast-Release (refined) Carbohydrates (pastries, puddings, manufactured sweets)
- No Shellfish (because of its high nuclein content)
- No Smoking (or tobacco in any form)
- No 'Junk' Beverages (carbonated sodas, etc.)
- No Apple Juice (too high in glucose)
- No Distilled Water

Some of the most important anti-cancer nutrients targeted in this serious work follow, along with an explanation of the work they perform within the body.

BETA-CAROTENE — This important element is a *precursor* of Vitamin A. In other words, the body uses beta-carotene to manufacture Vitamin A. Unlike Vitamin A, research has shown that beta-carotene does not harm the liver. With their important content of beta-carotene, new research indicates that carrots may have preventive and even curative powers in the case of cancer, particularly of the lungs. The cancer-preventive properties of beta-carotene are stronger than those of Vitamin A itself. The powerful difference between the two is that beta-carotene carries a mysterious type of live electrical charge, while Vitamin A does not. Another important difference is that beta-carotene has little harmful effect on the liver.

As both a preventive and an active cancer treatment, beta-carotene has been shown to effectively destroy the cancer cell's protective layer of mucus, opening it to the body's natural defense mechanisms. Proponents of beta-carotene predict reductions in the rate of certain forms of cancer for those who regularly include carrots in their diet (up to 80 percent of cancer in the lungs and bronchia, and up to 55 percent in cancer of the colon). Carrots are the single most important source of beta-carotene in nature. This common garden vegetable is considered the first line of defense as a cancer preventive of the highest order.

It is important to note that beta-carotene is fat-soluble and can only be absorbed and assimilated by the body in the presence of a fatty emulsion. The essential fatty acids the body requires are present in trace amounts in butter and cream, but a daily regimen which includes linseed oil and cottage cheese may be a healthier way to ingest these fats.

Raw carrot juice is considered a natural solvent for all ulcerous and cancerous conditions. Many naturopathic doctors suggest that smokers and those with a family history of cancer may benefit by adding a cup of raw carrots or freshly squeezed carrot juice to their daily diet. Some authorities believe the preventive powers of this dietary supplement may also apply to ulcers.

SKIN DISCOLORATION — It is not the beta-carotene or the orange coloring of carrots which tints the skin. You don't turn 'green' after eating green vegetables or 'red' after eating beets or 'orange' after eating carrots (or squash or apricots). An intensive treatment with carrots may tend to impart a yellowish-orange tint to the skin. If this happens to you, rejoice! The condition is temporary and shows that so many toxins are being leached out of the body that the overflow is being released through the pores of the skin.

The elements in carrots assist in detoxifying and cleansing the liver, one of the body's most important organs. If the normal eliminative passageways (intestines and urinary tract) are insufficient to carry it all away, the remainder is released through the skin. As a matter of fact, the skin itself is the largest eliminative organ of the body. (The wonders of beta-carotene are also targeted in Chapter 4.)

CHOLINE & METHIONINE — Laboratory studies confirm that a diet deficient in choline and methionine fosters the development of liver cancer. (A.K. Ghoshal and E. Farber: "The Induction of Resistant Hepatocytes during Initiation of Liver Carcinogenesis with Chemicals in Rats Fed a Choline-Deficient Methionine-Low Diet," *Carcinogenesis* Volume 4:801-804, 1983). In this landmark experiment, the researchers fed young, healthy male rats a diet (peanut meal and soya protein) which was low in choline and methionine for up to two years. Of the 45 rats fed the deficient diet, over half exhibited liver cancer (hepatocellular carcinoma). In startling contrast, not one of the rats in the control group given a choline supplement developed cancer. The scientists noted that liver cell necrosis began within just four to five *days* after feeding the deficient diet, followed by a period of very rapid hepatocyte (liver cancer cell) proliferation.

This effect was noted as long ago as 1961 by I.C. Wells and C.N. Remy. ("Inhibition of De Novo Choline Biosynthesis by 2-Amino-2-methyl-1-propanol," *Arch Biochemistry Biophysics*

Volume 95: 389-399, 1961.) Wells and Remy showed that inhibiting choline synthesis fostered the development of cancer. A diet deficient in choline and methionine (dietary methyl) clearly predisposes animals to liver cancer, even when an external cancer-producing agent is not present.

However, because a choline/methionine deficiency produces free radicals which damage DNA over the long-term, further tests are necessary to find out if the increased incidence of cancer exhibited by animals on a choline/methionine deficient diet is caused by the deficiency itself or by the damaged DNA.

GARLIC — As a cancer-fighter, garlic has shown amazing properties. Building on early studies which showed that malignant cells did not produce cancer when injected into laboratory animals — *if the tumor cells were first saturated with an active garlic extract* — Japanese scientists have injected mice with an anti-cancer vaccine consisting of live tumor cells soaked in garlic extract. Fourteen days after the mice were 'vaccinated' against cancer, the researchers injected the mice with live cancer cells. Not one mouse died and not one developed a malignancy. In contrast, the mice which served as the control group (which were not protected with the garlic-based anti-cancer vaccine) all developed cancer on schedule and all died within a 30-day period.

Dr. Mei Xing of the Shandong Medical College (Shandong, China) says that the regular consumption of garlic can lower the incidence of stomach cancer by inhibiting the formation of nitrites and nitrosamines, known to cause cancer in animals. In his 1981 study, Dr. Xing determined that the human volunteers involved in his research who took just one-third ounce of garlic showed significantly reduced nitrite levels within just four hours of ingestion. He says, "My study shows that garlic reduces the concentration of nitrite in the human stomach and may thus be considered a protective factor against the development of stomach (gastric) cancers."

Garlic has been used effectively by healers for over 5,000 years. History tells us that the ancients had a special regard for the health-promoting properties of this pungent herb. The scientists of today confirm that garlic has antiseptic, antibacterial, antifungal, and bacteriostatic properties. Modern researchers name garlic an amazing natural remedy for some forms of heart-disease, high blood pressure, diabetes, dysentery, pneumonia, and yeast infections. Regular use improves the immune system, normalizes the metabolic rate (thereby assisting in a weight-loss program), and promotes high energy levels.

SELENIUM — Selenium is an important element currently under investigation around the world as a possible aid to a healthy heart. Many heart patients who have fallen victim to a cardiac arrest or cardiac infarction have been shown to be deficient in selenium. Respected authorities believe selenium affords strong protection against cancer as well.

However, it has become difficult to take in enough selenium in the average diet. Soil studies show that many food-producing areas of the world lack selenium in their growing fields. If the nutrient is not available in the soil, it cannot be present in the food. A selenium deficiency is very common among the populations of the civilized world.

MAGNESIUM — A 10-year long German study has shown that patients taking magnesium (aspartate and orotate) therapy for heart disease have a 20 percent less incidence of cancer than occurs in the normal population mix. This research validates the observation that in regions where the drinking water is high in magnesium, there is a much lower rate of both cancer and heart disease.

Magnesium is known to enrich the body's immune defense system by assisting in the production of antibodies and strengthening the white blood cells. Magnesium is helpful to many other functions which maintain normal cell development as well. Since a malignancy is caused by abnormal cell development, it's easy to see why magnesium is a necessary cancer preventive.

A diet which includes a lot of whole-grains, fruits, and vegetables should supply sufficient magnesium for healthy functioning. Authorities say that a dangerously low level of magnesium is rare, but can occur. For instance, a junk-food diet, chronic diarrhea, or a condition which interferes with proper assimilation of nutrients can set the stage for a magnesium deficiency.

SODIUM — Although sodium is rarely found in the makeup of a normal cell, the abnormal cancerous cell pumps sodium into itself. When a cell goes haywire and becomes malignant, it loses the calcium lining of its inner membranes, with magnesium and potassium also being lost. With the loss of calcium, the cell loses its normal defense capabilities. By absorbing sodium, the cancer cell places itself beyond the body's normal defenses.

The blood analyses of cancer patients commonly show that not only the malignancy, but the blood cells themselves are overloaded with sodium. A promising theory suggests that removing the sodium (desodification) from the cancer cells would open them once more to the body's immune system defenses. But what substance can modern medicine offer to selectively remove the sodium from the cancer cells? The answer to this problem may yet come from a killer who lives in the depths of the oceans.

CURRENTLY IN RESEARCH

SQUALENE — In the human body and in all animals, cancer rarely finds a home in the cartilage. But the cartilage of the shark's fin is even more resistant to cancer than human cartilage. In fact, as a species, sharks appear to have a built-in protection against cancer, and not just in their fin cartilage either. A study conducted under the auspices of the Smithsonian Institute in Washington, D.C. discovered only one malignant tumor in 25,000 sharks!

The shark secretes certain substances (taurine and isaethionic acid) in its liver which constantly recycle the high salt concentration of its environment back into the sea. In current medical practice, taurine is often prescribed for both migraine headaches and epilepsy. The shark's anticancer potential is incredibly high because it is in a constant process of desodification.

The shark has yet another method of suppressing cancer. Along with its ability to eliminate sodium, the shark produces an oily substance called squalene. Squalene is produced in large quantities in the shark's liver and is also found in smaller amounts in both cod liver oil and olive oil. Researchers believe that squalene restores the vital electrostatic balance which is lost when a cell turns cancerous. Once the balance is restored by the squalene, the body's defense system can identify, attack, and destroy the malignancy.

DHEA — Dehydroepiandrosterone (DHEA) levels in the blood apparently play a protective role against the development of cancer. It has been determined that when DHEA levels in the blood rise to a value of more than 3.3 mg, a cancer tumor goes into remission. Squalene appears to stimulate the body's own production of DHEA. It is known that approximately 60 percent of the population contains sufficient natural DHEA to be protected from cancer. Of the remaining 40 percent deficient in DHEA, it is theorized that more than half (22 percent) will die from cancer.

ALDEHYDES — The 'bitter almond' (Laetrile/Mandelonitrile) substances exert a gene-repairing effect on cancer cells. These substances include amygdalin, prunasin, cassavin, ficin, and the synthetic mandelonitril compounds. Benzaldehyde (one of the constituents of Laetrile) has been shown to have a very positive effect against cancer cells. The excellent experimental and clinical results achieved in Japan with benzaldehyde treatments were published by the National Cancer Institute as long ago as 1980.

Various forms of aldehyde cancer therapy have been practiced in Germany at the Paracelsus Hospital in Hannover for more than 15 years. A respected head nurse with many years of experience working with cancer patients at this prestigious institution says of the 'bitter almond' substances, "Among all forms of medical cancer treatment, including poisonous chemotherapy, this is still the best method."

RUBIDIUM & CESIUM — Both are nontoxic elements shown to be absorbed by a cancer cell. Once absorbed, they neutralize the harmful hydrogen ions present in the malignancy. Studies indicate that this treatment has a positive effect even when a cancer growth has attained considerable volume, but primarily assists the body's own immune system. These elements should therefore be administered early, before the defenses of the body have been damaged beyond repair.

UREA — Urea is a natural product of metabolized protein long used in medicine as a diuretic and in the diagnosis of kidney function. Urea therapy is considered inexpensive, harmless, and can be used for a long period. Results achieved at the Greek Cancer Clinic as far back as the early 1970s show that urea has strong antiviral properties and is therefore effective against viral-induced malignancies, such as liver cancer (hepatitis B) and oral tumors (herpes virus).

As a powerful diuretic, urea has been shown to detoxify the body by eliminating cancer degradation byproducts. The Greek studies published in 1974 list several case histories of cancer patients then in remission after receiving between 10 and 18 grams of urea daily.

ASSISTING INTERNAL DEFENSE MECHANISMS

STEROIDS — Certain lymphocytes (white blood cells) play a very important part in the defense systems of the body. Lymph cells function efficiently only when they are present in sufficient quantity. In order to possess the ability to inactivate a cancerous cell, lymphocytes require special steroids: *thymosterine* and *tumosterone.* In order to manufacture tumosterone, the body must first manufacture its precursor, thymosterine. And, in order to be able to manufacture the precursor thymosterine, the body requires Vitamin D2. Prednisone (but no other cortisone) is also a precursor of thymosterine. The steroids thymosterine and tumosterone are both activated by the thymus gland. A healthy thymus gland is absolutely vital to an efficiently functioning immune system.

It is believed that tumosterone moves directly into the nucleus of the malignant cell via the lymph and inactivates it. However, this can only occur if a lymphocyte with sufficient tumosterone has identified and attached itself to the cancer cell.

German researchers have broken down tumosterone chemically and have succeeded in identifying the final metabolite of this protective element as 7-beta-hydroxy-cholsterol. This means that tumosterone can now be produced in a laboratory.

SHEEP LICE — Sheep are extremely resistant to cancer, possibly because their wool-fat has been shown to be especially rich in tumosterone. An old-country cure for viral hepatitis has been practiced in Germany for centuries. It consists of eating sheep lice. This is just one more demonstration of a folk medicine strongly rooted in what we now know to be scientific fact.

THE IMMUNE SYSTEM — Although it is difficult to stimulate the functioning of the thymus gland directly, science can provide elements which assist the immune system. A continuing intake of bromelaine, abundant in pineapples, may be a useful aid to the immune system and is considered an excellent cancer-preventive as well. Gamma-globulin, zinc-aspartate, manganese-aspartate, and molybdenum (abundant in cauliflower), are considered helpful. It has been noted that zinc enhances the body's defenses against cancer and exerts a pronounced preventive effect. But, caution must be observed. Once a malignant tumor has become established, zinc may increase its rate of growth.

ANTITUBERCULOSIS VACCINE — Over twenty years ago, researchers discovered that an injection of the antituberculosis vaccine BCG (Calmette-Guerin bacillus) can activate two or three different defense procedures of the white blood corpuscles. Clinical trials showed that these internal defenses can be dramatically effective, even against advanced cancer. The use of the vaccine demands particular care, however. Unless the body's immune system is still functioning, the vaccine may shut it down entirely.

AT INCREASED RISK

Certain whole segments of the population are, on average,

at increased risk of developing some type of cancer within their lifetimes. For instance, employment in the rayon industry carries a higher cancer risk, just as miners risk developing black lung. Predicting who will and who will not develop a malignancy within any given group of persons is not an exact science because so many diverse factors influence health.

However, the following information deserves your close attention. You just might find that you or someone you love is in a high-risk group without even being aware of it. Identifying high-risk groups is the first step to assisting these groups in lowering their risk. This very vital information is unknown to most of the American public.

BLOOD TYPE A — Cancer cells develop a defense mechanism of their own by surrounding themselves with a camouflaging layer of mucus. This protective outer layer makes it difficult for the body's own defenses to recognize a malignant cell and they hesitate to attack it.

Those of us with blood type A are at particular risk of developing cancer at some time in our lives because cancerous cells have a marked resemblance to blood type A cells. The defense system present in blood group A is not efficient in idenifying cancer cells and is very slow to attack, thereby giving the cancer a better chance of developing.

German research has documented this problem. Blood type A represents 43 percent, less than half, of the German population. But a whopping 77 percent, more than three-quarters, of the cancer victims in that nation are blood type A. At the opposite end of the scale, the study showed that only 19 percent of Germany's cancer patients are blood type O, but blood type O carriers represents the highest percentage of the general population.

Clearly, blood type A (and AB) carriers should incorporate all the preventive measures known into their lifestyles as quickly as possible in order to reduce their risk of developing cancer.

THE HEREDITY FACTOR — A comforting statistic comes from A.G. Knudson, M.D., Ph.D., of the Fox Chase Cancer

Center (Philadelphia, Pennsylvania). This eminent scientist received the prestigious Scientific Achievement Award given by the American Cancer Society (Philadelphia Division) in 1984. Dr. Knudson says, "I'd estimate that about five percent of all cancers are purely heredity. These include certain childhood cancers and melanomas."

Dr. Knudson points out that some genetic defects have been identified as promoting the development of cancer in children. Cancer of the eye (retinoblastoma) is caused when a portion of the chromosome 13 is missing. A malformation of chromosome 8 causes Wilms' tumor. Malignant melanomas (cancerous moles) also appear to run in families. Dr. Knudson says it's important to realize that true "cancer families" are rare. He says, "Cancer families tend to inherit the same cancer or cancers, and to get the disease at an early age. There is one family in which 50 percent of the members develop the same kind of kidney cancer. That's very different from having an uncle who got lung cancer, a sister with breast cancer, and a mother with stomach cancer."

However, statistics do show that a woman whose mother or sister had breast cancer has a greater chance of developing breast cancer herself. And, says Dr. Knudson, some other cancers (colon, ovarian, nervous system) appear to have a genetic basis as well.

THE FAMILY AT RISK — It has long been noted that being born into a cancer-prone family appears to increase your risk of developing a malignancy at some time in your life. The American Institute for Cancer Research has begun an all-out offensive to discover why cancer seems to run in certain families.

The research has zeroed in on one particular oncogene called the Ha-*ras* gene. The term *oncogene* comes from the Greek word 'oncos' or tumor. Scientists theorize that oncogenes are present in all cells and believe their function is to regulate cell growth. Because cancer cells grow abnormally, learning what factor regulates normal cell growth is vitally important. Once the growth factor is identified, medical science may be able to develop a procedure to control the abnormal proliferation of cancer cells.

When viewed under a powerful electronic microscope, the Ha-*ras* gene reveals as many as 20 distinct different patterns. In an intensive study of this particular oncogene, both cancer patients and those in the control group were shown to carry four of the most common patterns. Of the sixteen less common Ha-*ras* patterns, 12 were found only in cancer patients.

This important research indicates that persons carrying the Ha-*ras* gene in one of the 12 suspect configurations are at higher risk of contracting cancer than their brothers and sisters who may not have inherited one of the problem patterns. Science may soon be able to perform a simple blood test to determine your genetic risk of developing a malignancy.

If you carry one of the Ha-*ras* genes commonly found in cancer patients, it does not automatically follow that you will absolutely develop cancer. Being forewarned is forearmed. What this means is that you should immediately take all possible steps to reduce your risk from outside factors. Although you cannot control your genetic inheritance, you can incorporate preventive measures into your lifestyle.

GEOPATHOGENIC ZONES

EARTH DISTURBANCES — What exactly are *geopathogenic* zones, probably a term new to most, if not all, of the American public? An examination of the word itself provides the explanation. *Geo* comes from the Greek and means 'the earth.' *Pathogenic* is defined as 'disease producing.' *What?* Are there then certain zones of the earth which foster the development of disease?

Unfortunately, the answer appears to be *yes*. As long ago as 1920, the world-renowed German surgeon and oncologist Dr. Sauerbruch advised his cancer patients not to return to their homes if they were in a geopathogenic zone. Research into the possibility of low-frequency electrical disturbances deep within the earth increasing the risk of cancer to those who live in the vicinity began seriously over twenty years ago by Dr. Ernst Hartmann of Eberbach, Germany.

In the beginning, Dr. Hartmann's theory was ridiculed by orthodox medicine, and is still rejected today by most cancer authorities. But science has now determined that even a very weak electromagnetic pulse (between 5 and 25 Hz) can produce cancer cells. These extremely low frequencies (ELF) are active in geopathogenic zones. The major cause of these harmful ELF is the underground water flowing beneath the surface of the earth. The veins and arteries carrying the life-sustaining water supplies of the world produce these dangerous low frequencies, which, in theory at least, foster the development of cancer in those living above them.

Further documentation comes from Dr. Nieper who reports the following as a result of his own research and continuing observation of the cancer victims he himself treats: "According to studies I initiated, at least 92 percent of all the cancer patients I examined have remained for long time periods — especially with respect to their sleeping place—in geopathogenic zones. In my opinion, it is essential that tumor patients, as well as patients suffering from multiple sclerosis, be apprised of this information and depart geopathogenic zones."

There are certain manufactured devices available which are purported to *shield* the user from the damaging effects of the geopathogenic zones. Shielding devices are not effective. However, there are some devices which can, but only in part, *neutralize* the harmful ELF. One such device, called the 'North-South Rectifier,' is manufactured by the Henry Weber Company, Switzerland and another comes from Eberbach in Germany. At this writing, no effective ELF neutralizing devices are available in the U.S.

ELECTRICAL FIELDS

FRIEND TURNED FOE — Substantiating even further the harmful effect of certain electrical fields is the fact that persons working in electric transformer stations have a higher incidence of leukemia. Research originating at the University of Colorado corroborates the suspicion that people living in the vicinity of powerful electric mains suffer a higher incidence of cancer than the general population.

Another factor which is not well-known in the U.S. is the damaging effects of alternating current. According to German studies, when electric blankets, heating pads, massage units, and the like are activated by alternating current, the ELF waves which radiate from these commonly used items inactivate the body's electrostatic filtering system, which normally keeps the urinary tract passages bacteria-free.

Experienced (and aware) oncologists have observed that from the end of August until the first cold frosty nights of the winter season, the body's immune defense capacity is reduced by up to 30 percent. There is a documented and dramatic increase in the rate of growth of any malignancy in the body during this time of year. Around August 28th, the planets in the solar system pass through a dense system of magnetic fields. Some researchers theorize that certain electromagnetic factors thus created contribute to a drop in the body's defense mechanisms. This effect continues until the planets move on in early January.

During the damp months of autumn and continuing until the first hard freeze of winter, any mother will tell you that her family is more subject to sore throats, coughs, colds, and flu. This phenomenon, long recognized, is at least partially due to the fact that the first freeze destroys airborne bacteria. However, now that science has determined that the immune system is not working at full capacity during the planetary configurations that occur during this period, researchers are taking a hard look at the possibility that electromagnetic pulses reaching the earth should figure into their calculations.

TEMPERATURE CONTROL — Another comfort of modern technology which can become a potential health hazard is the American practice of turning up the thermostat. Of particular importance to all of us, especially cancer patients, is the news that experiments have shown that the body's immune defense system becomes sluggish and its efficiency drops drastically at temperatures over approximately 64.5 degrees F. (18 degrees C.).

Perhaps my readiness to accept the effects of the planets on man stems from learning the proper phases of the moon for planting from my grandfather. Or perhaps it's the memory of my grandmother and her unwavering belief in the importance of assisting the body through natural dietary means to work at optimum efficiency. But can't help but observe that orthodox medicine seems determined to alter chemically (or cut out) rather than assist naturally by recommending the proper foods and supplements which are known to strengthen the body's immune defenses.

FLUORIDE IS POISON

Fluoride is another avoidable carcinogen. It is a documented fact that as little as one-tenth of an ounce of fluoride can cause death, yet all over the country, fluoride is routinely added to city water supplies as a dental caries (cavity) preventive. Statistics from the National Academy of Sciences indicate that U.S. industries pump over 100,000 tons of fluoride waste into the atmosphere every year and dump even more (an estimated 500,000 tons) into our waters. *Yes, fluoride is an industrial waste product* occurring in the production of aluminum. And, yes, it is this same industrial waste that is used to fluoridate our drinking water.

According to the 1983 *U.S. Pharmacopeia Volumes on Drug Information,* the following clinical signs of fluoride poisoning occur with alarming frequency among people ingesting tablets containing the amount of fluoride found in just 1 to 2 pints of fluoridated water: Black stool (tar-like), bloody vomiting, diarrhea, faintness, nausea, shallow breathing, stomach pain or cramps, tremors, unusual excitement, unusual increase in saliva, watery eyes, weakness, constipation, loss of appetite, bone involvement (aches and pains), skin rash, sores (mouth, lips), stiffness, weight loss, mottling of teeth (white, brown, or black discolorations).

FLUORIDE POISONINGS — A town in Kizilcaoren, Turkey has been dubbed *Das Dorf der jungen Greise,* "the village where people age before their time," by the German researchers studying this phenomenon. All the inhabitants of this area suffer from premature aging. Between the ages of 30 and 40, they develop the wrinkled skin typical of the normal

60 year old; young women give birth to dead babies after pregnancies of only 4 months duration; men of 30 are impotent; all suffer from a severe weakness of the musculoskeletal structure and walking is impossible without the support of a stick. Sick livestock slaughtered for food show diseased livers.

The slow and insidious poisoning of the villagers was uncovered by a dentist who noted the typical mottling (brown discoloration) of extreme fluoride poisoning on the teeth of all children over the age of 7 and complete discoloration of teeth in teenagers. Most adults in the village had just a few affected teeth remaining. When notified of this phenomenon, the medical staff at the University Clinic of Eskisehir, Turkey conducted an intensive investigation. Their report concluded that, on top of the reproductive difficulties and dental involvement pervading the population, "Every single inhabitant of Kizilcaoren suffers from a bone disease with symptoms including thickening of the ankles, stiffened joints, and abnormal growth of bone substance."

In neighboring Turkish villages where water is drawn from different sources, normal health prevails. But in Das Dorf der jungen Greise, water from the village well was found to contain an extremely high naturally-occurring fluoride concentration of 5.4 ppm (parts per million).

THE FLUORIDE/CANCER CONNECTION

THE IMMUNE SYSTEM — Scientists at the Seibersdorf Research Center in Austria have reported that as little as 1 ppm fluoride slows down the vitally important DNA repair enzyme activity of the immune system. It has long been noted that the higher incidence of cancer among older persons is directly related to the proven decline in the ability of the immune system to repair defective DNA components.

Numerous laboratory studies have shown that fluoridated water (at concentrations as low as 1 ppm) can cause serious genetic and chromosomal damage in plants, animals, and humans. Using bone marrow and testes cells, a U.S. geneticist has demonstrated that the degree of chromosomal damage increases proportionately as the fluoride content of the water increases. It is important to note that abnormal sperm cells which have been damaged by fluoride poisoning can lead to serious birth defects and certain metabolic disorders that can be passed on from generation to generation.

Using the same level of fluoride commonly put into U.S. water supplies, scientists at the Nippon Dental College in Japan have determined that this minute amount of fluoride is capable of transforming normal cells into cancer cells. At a meeting of the Japanese Association of Cancer Research in Osaka in 1982, the researchers reported, "Last year at this meeting we showed that sodium fluoride, which is being used for the prevention of dental caries, induces chromosomal aberrations and irregular synthesis of DNA. This year, we report our finding that a malignant transformation of cells is induced by sodium fluoride."

As incredible as it may seem, research sponsored by the American Cancer Institute as long ago as 1963 clearly showed that even very low levels of fluoride increased the incidence of melanotic tumors in experimental laboratory animals by a frightening 12 to 100 percent. Similar types of transformations of normal cells to potentially cancerous cells have been observed in humans.

Polish scientists working at the Pomeranian Medical Academy have published reports that as little as 0.6 ppm fluoride produces chromosomal damage in human white blood cells, the important defensive cells of the immune system.

SURPRISING FINDINGS

If some of this information comes as a surprise to you, we invite you to consider it carefully and incorporate whatever seems good and logical into your own lifestyle. Many of the preventive measures suggested are both inexpensive and simple. For instance, by merely adding carrot juice to your daily regimen, you will be providing your body with beta-carotene, an incredibly powerful cancer preventive.

I'll drink a toast to your health tomorrow morning at breakfast with my morning carrot juice! I recommend it highly.

Recent research has found other common substances that are cancer-linked. One of the most used and abused food items is refined sugar.

SUGAR AND SUGAR SUBSTITUTES

White sugar has almost no nutritional value, but the average American consumes about 60 pounds of the stuff each year. Dr. Linus Pauling wrote in 1981 that Americans over the past 75 years, have upped their sugar consumption by 50 percent. At the same time, their consumption of fruits, vegetables and whole grains has dropped by 40 percent. It's not surprising that many "well-fed" Americans have nutrition deficiencies.

Research shows that cancer cells thrive in a sugar-rich environment. Those interested in lowering their cancer risk should also lower their sugar consumption, or cut it out altogether.

Many calorie or nutrition-conscious consumers opt instead for artificial sweeteners. Aspartame, mass-marketed as "NutraSweet®," is the latest wave of artificial sweeteners.

NUTRASWEET® OR ASPARTAME

NutraSweet® is made from aspartic acid and phenylalanine, chemicals that break down into amino acids inside the body. What the ads don't tell you is that phenylalanine is toxic to brain tissue. It causes alarming reactions in some humans - symptoms like dizziness, headaches, epileptic-like seizures, eye pain and bleeding and menstrual problems. Early complaints lodged with the product manufacturer took weeks to be reported to the Food and Drug Administration.

The FDA agrees that a small percentage of the population may be sensitive to aspartame. Those diagnosed with inherited phenylketonuria should avoid the substance, which can cause amino acids to accumulate in the body. Because NutraSweet® is still new on the market, the FDA warns pregnant women to curb their consumption of the chemical.

Its long-term effect on unborn children is unknown.

Despite its known health hazards, aspartame is still widely marketed. Several studies performed at Massachusetts Institute of Technology continue to show an alarming seizure risk to those who use the substance regularly, especially women between the ages of 20 and 40. But because MIT uses reporting methods different from the FDA's, the federal agency refuses to consider the institute's studies.

Another aspartame study was done in 1993 at Northeastern Ohio University College of Medicine in Youngstown. Patients with mood disorders were found to have major reactions to the sweetener: symptoms like severe eye pain, (including one case of retinal detachment), nervousness, memory difficulties, nausea and depression. Patients' reactions were severe enough that the medical school's Institutional Review Board had the doctors discontinue the experiments.

The study was not deemed broad enough to cause the FDA to ban the product, but those with mood disorders are now advised to avoid NutraSweet®.

Use of NutraSweet® has not been linked to cancer formation, but anyone interested in staying healthy may be well-advised to avoid this sugar substitute, as well as Saccharine, which does create cancer cells in laboratory rats.

ALCOHOL

Men who drink some forms of Scotch and Bourbon whiskies have a greater incidence of mouth and throat cancers.

People who drink to excess have more nutritional problems than other group of Americans. They develop infections quickly, and have a harder time getting over them. In addition to the common liver ailments, alcohol can damage the brain, nervous, lymphatic and venous systems.

But how much is too much? The United States Department of Health and Human Services recommends you limit yourself to two alcoholic drinks per day. Many doctors say that's still too much. (A drink is defined as one 12-ounce beer, one 5-ounce glass of wine or a mixed drink containing 1.5 ounces of spirits.)

Shaw and Lieber, nutritional researchers, reported in a professional journal "Nutritional Support of Medical Practice" that alcoholics get about 20 percent of their calorie intake from alcohol, not food. Alcohol has no nutritional value, but frequently gives the drinker a "full" feeling. This doesn't always leave much room for food.

Alcohol abusers therefore suffer a number of vitamin deficiencies, which leaves them susceptible to cancer-causing agents and tumor development. Medical evidence dating back to the 18th century suggests that overindulgence directly inhibits the body's immune system. With repeated alcohol abuse, the drinker's white blood cell count goes down, which creates the risk of tuberculosis, viral infections and cancer.

The International Agency for Research on Cancer says that heavy drinkers have higher-than-normal rates of cancers of the mouth, throat, esophagus, larynx, bladder, breast and liver. Many alcoholic beverages naturally contain urethane, a known chemical carcinogen. This is not an additive; it forms as part of the fermenting process that creates wine, beer and "hard liquor."

WHAT TO DO

If you drink, limit yourself to two drinks each day.

If you are pregnant or breastfeeding, do not drink.

If you find yourself consuming more than two drinks each day, cut down immediately. Find out what motivates you to drink: perhaps a support group or counselor can help.

Above all, eat a nutritionally sound diet. Don't let alcohol become your "food." Remember that alcohol acts as a poison to your body. It has no food value at all.

Chapter XII
Healthy Living
A Summary of What's Good & What's Not

GOOD FOODS

LINSEED OIL — is at the very top of the list of good foods. This dietary fat is so vitally important to your health that we have devoted a great deal of space to explaining exactly what the essential fatty acids (linoleic and linolenic) do for you. We have explored the ways that linseed oil and cottage cheese, an excellent source of the sulphur-based proteins that activate the essential fatty acids, can dissolve tumors and restore even a terminal cancer victim to health. If you are skeptical of the wonders of crude linseed oil, please review Chapter 6 again.

We hate to remind you of the fact that the majority of U.S. brands of linseed oil generally don't measure up. There is however a product formulated from Europe that is from the first pressing of the seeds. You can trust that the essential fatty acids are present in rich abundance in virgin *C-Leinomed*™ (Linomed).

GARLIC — Garlic is mentioned several times within these pages as being a particularly healthy food. It has been used medically for centuries against congestion, circulatory problems, heart disease and more. As a powerful cancer preventive and therapeutic, garlic shows great promise.

I can't imagine anyone who doesn't enjoy this pungent herb, but if you just plain don't like garlic, you'll be interested in the newest garlic formulation to hit the market. This new garlic product is a new biologically active garlic preparation. Using the very latest technology, garlic cloves are harvested and processed straight from the garden to capture and preserve all the volatile oils and natural elements. The end result is a caplet containing all the vital health-promoting activity of this pungent herb. Studies comparing this method of processing with freshly harvested garlic show that the active constituents in both are the same. This new exciting and enriched Ivan Robroff's original formula from Bulgaria contains hawthorn, hops, rutin, in an exclusive formulation which synergistically potentiates the scientifically documented healthful properties of the garlic itself.

Hawthorn promotes blood circulation through the coronary arteries and serves to maintain normal blood pressure. Garlic benefits the entire alimentary tract, especially where indigestion tends to occur. It helps normalize the blood pressure, particularly when fluctuation arises and acts on the cholesterol deposits in the blood vessels, thereby preventing the risk of arteriosclerosis. Hops helps to cleanse the blood, tone up the liver, stimulate a sluggish gallbladder and increase the flow of bile. It has a calming effect on the nervous system as it removes restlessness and promotes sleep. Rutin is a good source of bioflavonoids and helps the body utilize vitamin C. It strengthens fragile blood vessels and helps prevent their recurrent bleeding.

CARROTS — There's so much hard scientific evidence showing that the beta-carotene content of carrots alone qualifies this ancient root vegetable as an efficient cancer preventive and one which assists in the therapeutic treatment of fatty degeneration as well, that the point can hardly be argued. Carrots contain many important vitamins and minerals, making them exceptionally valuable nutritionally. As a raw addition to a salad, they offer a good quantity of sulphur-rich amino acids. A number of the vital alkaline elements are present in carrots in perfectly balanced proportions. These elements aid the body in many important functions, including the efficient assimilation of the essential fatty acids.

We remind you again that beta-carotene is fat-soluble and can only be used by the body in the presence of a fatty emulsion. The essential fatty acids the body requires are present in trace amounts in butter and cream, but, as we have discussed at length, a daily regimen which includes linseed oil and cottage cheese is a much healthier way to ingest these

FIBER FOODS — The average daily intake of fiber in the westernized and industralized nations is around 4 grams. In the so-called uncivilized countries, the daily fiber intake hovers around 30 grams, precisely the amount health experts recommend. Conditions of the digestive system and intestinal tract common to our society include constipation, a national problem continuing to grow by astronomical proportions. Other disorders include cancer of the colon, diverticulosis and diverticulitis, diseases of the large intestine and rectum, and hemorrhoids. These conditions are uncommon in areas where fiber intake is high.

Two generations ago, our daily diet included a lot of what grandmother called 'roughage.' Grandmother served brown rice and cereal grains that were unmilled and unrefined, and she usually baked her own bread. She put a lot of raw vegetables fresh from the garden on the table, or cooked them with the skins on to 'save vitamins.' We enjoyed our fruits sun-warmed and ate them whole, ingesting a lot of healthy fiber in the bargain.

Today, fruits turn up as a jumble of bits and pieces in a can labeled 'fruit cocktail.' The fiber that was in the skin has been discarded. orange juice is now filtered and 'concentrated,' with all the sweet pulp removed. The pulp and white membrane that separates the sections, rich in fiber, has been thrown away. Today, we have to eat 16 slices of commercially baked white bread (made with hydrogenated oils, another warning sign) in order to consume the 30 grams of fiber contained in just 4 slices of whole-grain bread. Are you beginning to track the clues to the problem here?

Another important factor in favor of fiber is that it contains no calories, meaning that it can't go to your waist (or hips). Fiber passes through the body virtually unchanged. It supplies bulk needed by the intestines to remove body wastes with such haste that they don't have time to putrify and cause irreparable harm. (See Chapter 3 for a fast review of how fiber works as a cancer preventive.) However, a high fiber diet acts to leach some important minerals from the system and quickly excretes them. When adding fiber to your diet, make sure your diet also contains foods rich in calcium (dairy products, eggs, beans, cauliflower), magnesium (whole grains, vegetables, fruits), and zinc (milk, liver, shellfish, herring, wheat bran). (Note: As a powerhouse containing *all* essential nutrients, bee pollen is a good natural source of these three minerals.)

The recommendations are clear, but if your dietary habits are too firmly entrenched to make the necessary changes, a product called *Fibermed-7*™ may be your answer. Along with healthy natural herbal fiber, this important supplement contains a measure of calcium, magnesium, and zinc, precisely the minerals the body especially needs when additional fiber is added to the diet. With apple fiber, oat fiber, alfalfa, carob, apple pectin, arrow root, cellulose, dandelion root, marshmallow root, oat straw, slippery elm, and Chinese cinnamon, plus the vital minerals listed above, the ingredients in this product might have been selected by Mother Nature herself. In convenient caplet form, *Fibermed 7*™ has the rather pleasant taste of nature in the raw, and may be chewed for faster assimilation, if desired. This is the easy way to supplement your diet with healthy fiber.

Note: Although fiber itself has no caloric value, fiber-rich foods contain varying amounts of calories. For those on a weight-loss regimen, taking a fiber supplement might be the wiser course. For example, eating 4 slices of delicious whole-grain bread will easily supply the day's optimum amount of fiber, but there are times when eating this amount of bread will add some unwanted and unnecessary calories to the menu.

RAW FOODS — After the traditional Thanksgiving feast, a big Sunday dinner, or other heavy meal, we usually push back from the table, yawn, and feel so tired we're impelled to take a snooze. We put that tired feeling down to overeating, and that's part of it, but there's a further explanation. When we feed on cooked (dead) food, the body fights back. The stomach and intestinal tract reacts to the mass of cooked foods by rushing white blood cells to the scene and with swelling or bloating. The temperature in the localized area rises and develops a 'fever.' In case you didn't recognize this reaction, it is the same reaction the body exhibits in the presence of an infection *and* around a tumor.

Cooking destroys all the living digestive enzymes in food. The body is forced to secrete an extra supply of digestive enzymes in order to process the dead mass. Late-breaking research coming out of Europe tells us that the body reacts in the same way when just part of the meal is eaten cooked and part of the meal is eaten raw — *if* the cooked food is ingested first. However, if we first eat some raw foods before consuming the cooked portion of the meal, the reaction does not occur.

A very few foods are not good for us in their raw state. Raw potatoes are just not tasty, even though their nutritional value is high. Raw beans contain a protein-like substance *(phaseolin)* which can cause indigestion. Raw egg whites contain another protein-like element *(avidin)* which inhibits the absorption of important B vitamins. Avidin is destroyed in cooking. (If you enjoy a protein shake made in your blender, don't use raw eggs as part of the ingredients.)

But it's delightful to begin a meal with a big salad of leafy greens and raw vegetables. Make sure your salad contains shredded carrots, garlic, green (or red) bell peppers, hot peppers (if you like them), radishes, and onions along with dark green leafy 'lettuces.' Spinach is one of the best. Dress your salad with one of the linseed oil and cottage cheese based salad dressing recipes given in Chapter 7 and give your long-suffering stomach a rest!

BEE POLLEN — For a healthy helping of live enzymes, there's no better source than a high quality bee pollen. The golden granules of this nutritional sunshine from the beehive, when correctly handled, are richly enzyme active and a superior source of all the nutrients (amino acids, vitamins, minerals, essential fatty acids, hormones, carbohydrates, trace elements) required by the life processes. As a cancer fighter, bee pollen has been shown in scientifically controlled double-blind studies to inhibit the development of tumors. Also, cancer victims undergoing radiation therapy found the debilitating side-effects of this form of treatment were reduced and easier to bear when they were given bee pollen.

Our vote for the best bee pollen goes to a relative newcomer and is harvested in areas free of environmental contamination, such as some of the western states, and is cold processed to protect enzymatic activity, is a blended multi-source product, and is packaged to insure all properties remain active and potent. Some of the world's greatest health authorities say that pollen is nature's perfect food and is hailed as the hope for total youth, and so many people can greatly benefit from taking them daily. They are loaded with energy giving properties.

SUSPECT FOODS

SUGAR — When we eat food (carbohydrates), it is true that the body sorts out all the elements and eventually breaks down the constituents into simple sugars (glucose and fructose). *Glucose* is the major sugar present in blood and body tissues. This is an essential sugar in that all cells, especially brain cells, depend on glucose. But there is no RDA (Recommended Daily Allowance) for any kind of sugar, including glucose. We are not required to eat a measure of glucose every day. The specialized enzymes of the digestive tract are equipped to convert carbohydrates into the basic glucose the body needs. Glucose is released slowly into the bloodstream during the metabolic process, along with other needed nutrients.

One of the most common misconceptions today, fostered by some excellent advertising, is that white sugar (which is not glucose, but *sucrose*) provides quick energy and is a good food. The catch is that sugar is not absorbed and metabolized in the body in the same efficient way as complex carbohydrates are. When we eat sugar, it is rapidly absorbed and passed on to the liver where it is converted into triglycerides. The triglycerides are released into the bloodstream and end up being stored as fat deposits in the veins and tissues. Do we have to remind you that high cholesterol and triglyceride levels are implicated in the development of cancer, heart disease, and many other life-threatening conditions?

An intake of sugar also triggers the release of insulin by the pancreas. The insulin metabolizes the sugar rapidly in order to maintain normal blood-sugar levels. But the sugar is digested and assimilated so quickly that a lot of excess insulin (with a much longer half-life than sugar) continues racing around the bloodstream and is left with nothing to process. This is the big reason why sugar picks you up fast, but lets you down even faster. Sugar is not a source of sustained energy at all. The ingestion of large amounts of sugar over a long period of time places tremendous stress on the pancreas. Diabetes results when the pancreas is exhausted and loses its ability to synthesize insulin. Diabetes (and related side effects) ranks third (after heart disease and cancer) as a cause of death in America.

CHEMICAL FOOD ADDITIVES — You're having a few people in for the evening. In your best party snack bowls, you serve your guests some citric acid mixed with propylene glycol, a variety of glycerides, some butylated hydroxyanisole, butylated hydroxytoluene, propyl gallate, chemically-altered fats, and an excessive amount of sodium, plus, of course, a measure of dye and artifical flavoring. All this yucky stuff is part of the ingredients you usually find in a bag of corn chips. Still hungry?

As of 1983, the FDA had approved the use of more than 3,000 food additives. The number of additives listed as GRAS (Generally Regarded As Safe at a specified level) in 1983 totaled over 1,000. Today, some authorities estimate that as many as 7,000 chemicals appear in our foods.

The food industry spends over *20 billion dollars* every year on the chemical additives they put in our food. An educated guess is that each of us consumes over five pounds of chemical preservatives, stabilizers, dyes, artificial flavorings, and other additives each year without really thinking much about it.

These chemicals serve a variety of purposes. They act as bleaching agents, extenders, clarifiers, emulsifiers, softeners, thickeners, hydrogenators, curing agents, buffers, deodorizers, sprout inhibitors, fungicides, sweeteners, conditioners, antioxidants, fortifiers, drying agents, alkalizers, defoamers, firming agents, stabilizers, and preservatives.

We have to depend on the FDA to test and approve (or disallow) food additives. New substances are tested on lab animals and those that prove deadly within 24 hours to two weeks of ingestion are evaluated further. Another test is to determine what quantity of a substance must be ingested to kill half the animals during the experimental period. This is the test used to determine 'safe' levels of ingestion for humans.

Unfortunately, there is no established testing procedure to discover the effects of ingesting a *combination* of chemicals, something we do every day. Interestingly enough, the FDA itself has shown that consuming just *one-tenth* of the fatal amount (presumably a 'safe' level) of two different chemicals at the same time can result in death. It's impossible for science to establish 'safe' levels of ingestion of a potentially dangerous substance without knowing exactly what substances we might consume along with it.

Most food additives are nutritionally valueless. Additives are used mainly to make inferior foods cosmetically attractive, to make them 'convenient' to prepare, and to extend shelf life. *We really do know there's a better way to eat,* but the food industry mounts massive advertising campaigns to convince us otherwise. And we let ourselves be persuaded. Here's a quick review of some of the common food additives we eat every day:

BHA & BHT — Butylated hydroxyanisole (BHA) and butylated hydroxytoluene (BHT) are popular antioxidants which are used to prevent foods (in which the natural antioxidants have been refined out) from going rancid on the shelves over a long period. These petroleum-based chemicals have been banned in Great Britain and many other countries of the world, but the powerful food processors in the U.S. equate long shelf life with corporate profits. It's my guess that BHA and BHT will be with us for a long time. You'll find BHA and BHT in cereals, candy, gelatin, shortening, ice cream, dairy foods, processed meats, peanut butter, margarine, chewing gum, vegetable oils, dried fruits, meats, fish, salad dressings, most popular snack foods, and much more.

Lead — Canned meats and milk may become contaminated with lead (from the seal on the can), but we also take in lead unwittingly from toothpaste, aluminum foil, car exhausts, factory wastes, and other canned foods.

MSG — Monosodium glutamate has been around a long time. In 1968, researchers at Washington University determined that excessive intake damaged brain cells in lab animals. As a result of these findings, baby food manufacturers discontinued use of MSG. Just one-quarter teaspoon of MSG can upset the digestive processes and produces an allergic reaction in many infants.

Nitrates — In combination with nitrosamines, nitrates pose an unnecessary cancer risk. The American Cancer Society has recommended we sharply reduce our consumption of cured and processed meats (ham, bacon, sausage, hot dogs, cold cuts) because of their content of nitrates and nitrites. (For more, see Chapter 4.)

'ENRICHED' BREADS — Are you fooled by the word 'enriched' on that spongy supermarket bread? Here's the inside story:

Monostearates — Monostearates are classified as 'emulsifiers.' An emulsifier causes flour to absorb up to six times its own weight in water. In humans, it acts on tissues and cells and increases their absorption capacity. This means we are likely to absorb toxins and poisons at an accelerated rate. Laboratory animals fed monostearates developed diarrhea and ulcerations, bled internally all along the genito-urinary tract, and died within weeks. Studies show that monostearates cause cancer in rats.

Propionates — Propionates are used to slow down the growth of molds, making the bread appear fresh longer. Propionates (also a prime ingredient in ointments and powders for treating athlete's foot) are steam-processed from ethylene and carbon monoxide and interfere with the body's ability to assimilate calcium.

Inorganic Calcium — The synthetic form of calcium used to 'enrich' breads can't be assimilated by the body anyway.

Ammonium Chloride — Powdered soaps and detergents, antifreeze, and many breads contain this chemical. In bread making, it is used to ferment dough.

Potassium Bromate — Many home permanents contain potassium bromate; the label carries a warning not to drink it. In bread making, potassium bromate holds in air bubbles while the loaf is baking, providing the spongy texture.

Inorganic Iron — The form of iron (ferrum radactum) used to enrich most breads can't be assimilated or used by the body.

Chemically-Altered Fats — Most breads are made with hydrogenated or partially hydrogenated fats. (See Chapter 5.)

Refined Flour — With all its healthy fiber stripped away, and most vitamins and minerals eliminated in the refining process, the nutrient value of refined flour breads is questionable. Do we need to remind you that The American Cancer Society says fiber is an important part of the anticancer diet? A diet deficient in fiber promotes obesity. We overeat refined low-nutrient foods because the body tries desperately to secure the nutrients it needs to function. A high fiber diet also prevents constipation and related problems, such as hemorrhoids.

THE HAZARDS OF EATING OUT — Walk into any restaurant, tell the maitre d' (or manager) you're allergic to *sulfites,* ask if sulfites are in the foods they serve, and you'll probably be rewarded with a blank stare. Nowdays, most restauranteurs can tell you they don't cook with MSG, and many will say they don't use sulfites on their salad greens or fresh vegetables, but most are unaware of the sulfites in commercially processed foods.

Sulfites — Although asthmatics who ingest sulfites are at greater risk than most of us, about 25 percent of the complaints received by the FDA regarding sulfites come from persons who don't have a history of asthma. Symptoms of sulfite sensitivity include: severe respiratory distress, vomiting, nausea, diarrhea, abdominal pain and cramps, hives, unconsciousness and death. At least 20 deaths associated with sulfite consumption had been reported to the FDA by 1985.

In one or the other of its many disguises, sulfites function as preservatives and/or antioxidants. Some are used as bleaching agents for food starches, some are used in the manufacturing of cellophane, and some are used as sterilizing agents. Salad fixings are dipped or dusted with sulfites to preserve their fresh look and appetizing color.

Sulfites include a variety of sulfur-based additives (sulfur dioxide, sodium sulfite, sodium and potassium bisulfite, sodium and potassium metabisulfite). You'll find sulfites in baked goods, chip dips, dried fish, canned or dried fruits, juices, gelatin, potato products, salad dressings, relishes, sauces, gravies, sauerkraut, cole slaw, shellfish (fresh, frozen, canned), dried and canned soups, vegetables (frozen, dried, canned), vinegars, wine, beer, and cider.

It's hard to understand just how sulfites have assumed such importance. People have been baking for centuries without sulfites. People have been drying fish, vegetables, fruits, and even meats for centuries without sulfites. People have been eating shellfish for centuries without sulfites. People have been making wine, beer, and cider for centuries without adding sulfites. When I was a child, I remember my grandmother making sauerkraut (and many other cabbage dishes) without sulfites. The only reason sulfites are added to our foods today is to improve the look of inferior foods and extend the shelf life.

HERE'S HOW TO FIGHT BACK

Money talks. If enough of us simply stop buying over-processed foods over-laden with chemical additives (or with their original nutrients chemically altered into alien elements that the body doesn't recognize and can't metabolize), the food processors will get the message. Food processors are in business to make money. Health-food stores are picking up customers by leaps and bounds as more and more people become aware of the dangers of chemically-laced foods.

Organically-Grown — The producers of organically grown produce (and meats) are now being actively sought out by those 'in the know' who want to avoid the profusion of harmful chemicals creeping into the food chain courtesy of giant agribiz executives. These giant producers are more interested in bringing food animals to market size in a hurry, and in growing ever-larger food crops by taking advantage of chemical technology, than they are in producing nutritious food.

Yes, you do pay more for foods certified as being organically produced, and that's a large stumbling block for many of us. But, it might very well be a question of 'pay now' or 'pay later' in the form of increased medical bills.

As biochemists and medical science learn more about the workings of human cells and genetics, the far-reaching implications of this constant consumption of chemicals becomes truly alarming. It is frighteningly obvious that we don't know enough about the *cumulative* effects of food additives, and it may take many years (possibly generations) before the effects are fully manifested.

And this is exactly the way cancer (and other degenerative diseases) work. One single cell gone wrong can be the start. Over time (sometimes as long as 10 or 20 years), a slow growing malignancy develops until the symptoms finally become noticeable.

We can't blame all our health problems on the food industry. The law of supply and demand comes into play. If processed foods weren't selling (and we spend billions of dollars on them every year), the industry would immediately replace them with food items more to our liking. If the newest convenience food doesn't grab its share of our food dollars, it's gone. Market researchers know exactly what the consumer buys.

SHOPPING IN THE ENEMY CAMP — If you're armed with enough knowledge (and we're trying), you can safely shop for most of your food needs in a supermarket. But what you *must* do is learn to read labels.

Sugar — A reminder that sugar is in just about everything. Sugar contributes to diabetes and hypo/hyperglycemia. It provides nothing but empty calories that the body doesn't need or want. *You* may have trained your body to crave processed sweets, but it knows better. Try honey instead. *Note:* Honey is a natural sweet, but is even more strongly implicated in the development of dental decay than sugar. Why? Because of its viscosity, it clings to the teeth longer than sugar. (You should be brushing after every meal anyway.)

Cola Drinks — If you drop a human tooth into a cola, it begins to dissolve in just 48 hours.

Soft Drink Powders — These popular products are dyed chemicals with artificial flavors. The 'sugarless' varieties usually contain NutraSweet® .

Juices — I can't imagine why natural sweets have to be sugared. It's hard to find any juice (fruit or vegetable) in the supermarket that doesn't contain added sugar in some form, but it can be done. Read the label before you bring it home.

Fresh Produce — You're on safer ground here. The fresh produce in the supermarket hasn't been organically grown and may be lower in nutrients than products grown nature's way, but at least it isn't refined. Ask the produce manager if they use sulfites, and remember to watch out for irradiated foods. (See 'Nuked Foods' this chapter.) vegetables and fruits are rich in vitamins, mineral, nutrients, and fiber the mainstay of a healthy diet.

Whole-Grain Products — When buying breads (crackers, snacks) read the label carefully. Don't buy products made with refined flours or hydrogenated/partially hydrogenated oils. Whole wheat bread isn't necessarily made with the *whole* grain. Check the label to see if the bran (outer covering) and germ are in there.

246

Cereals — There are many cereal boxes to read, but do it. You'll really be surprised to find how few brands are made *with* the whole grain and *without* added sugar.

Meat, Fish, Poultry — Never buy any processed meats. Forget about frozen fish with a 'crispy' coating, but do enjoy fresh or frozen fillets (baked or poached). Skin poultry to reduce saturated fat consumption.

'NUKED' FOODS — *What* — In early 1986, the Federal Government approved the use of radiation to kill insects on fruits and vegetables. During this process, the food is chemically changed, but Radiation Technology, Inc. (Rockaway, New Jersey) tells us that the change in nutrient value is 'nominal.'

When — Irradiating of some pork products began a while back when the FDA approved a special petition from a pork packer. Because approval was sought by petition from an outside company, the FDA was not bound to publish proposed regulations and solicit consumer reaction. Critics had 30 days to protest, but not enough of us knew about it. You may have been eating irradiated pork since mid-1985 without knowing it.

Where — By the time you read this, even more irradiated products will be in supermarkets all over the country. By law, for the next two years, all foods thus treated must carry the words 'treated by radiation' (or 'irradiation') and must display the international symbol of this treatment.

The symbol is a broken circle with a small ball and two leaves in the middle. Watch for it. The only way you'll be able to tell if you are purchasing (and eating) radiated food is to spot the symbol. You can't see a difference and you can't taste a difference. The chemical disarrangment of the atoms and electrons in foods thus treated are both invisible and tasteless.

Irradiation Symbol

Certain fruits are targeted for processing with radiation. Peaches, strawberries, melons, nectarines, and papayas — the harvest of summer are the most likely candidates. We are told that 'nuked' fruits may be more expensive because the process is new. We are supposed to be thankful because they will last longer than their natural untreated cousins.

Why — Radiation does, we are assured, extend the shelf life of the foods thus treated. This undoubtedly will benefit the food industry, but what does it mean to the consumer? Unfortunately, no one knows. The process is too new for anyone to know exactly what the long term effects of eating 'nuked' foods might be.

WHY CONSUMER CONCERN IS JUSTIFIED — Some scientists and many health authorities say this process raises more questions than can be answered at the present time. We just don't know exactly what the chemical changes radiation causes in foods will do in the body. It has been determined that most of the x-rays used to bombard the food in this process do pass straight through without changing the intrinsic structure of the food itself. So far, so good. It's the rays that remain behind in the food that are causing concern.

URPs — True, these electrons do kill insects, destroy the bacteria that cause spoilage, and inhibit the ripening process to insure a longer shelf life. But they destroy certain natural bonds in the food and also bind with the natural elements to create entirely new chemical substances that Mother Nature never heard of. These newly created chemicals which are found to occur in radiation treated foods have been dubbed URPs (*unique radiolytic products*). Virtually nothing is known about them or their possible effects on health.

Concerned consumer groups like the Public Citizen Health Research Group (Washington, D.C.) point out that the only way to determine if the URPs are toxic or worse, cancer-causing, is by feeding these substances to laboratory animals in the usual long-term controlled testing procedures. To date, studies sponsored by the U.S. Department of Agriculture with foods exposed to high levels of radiation found some serious dangers to health, including damage to the testes (and testicular tumors), a decease in the number of offspring, and lowered survival rates.

Although studies have not shown that irradiated foods are safe, and current FDA policy requires extensive testing of food chemicals (which has not been done with radiated food), for some reason the Food & Drug Administration appears to be ignoring its own safety regulations in this case. The Health Research Group says that the FDA's decision to allow irradiation of foods is based on *estimates* of the amount of URPs which may be produced during processing, and not on actual scientific evidence. We are back to square one. No one really knows what effects radiated foods can or will have in the body.

Changes in Nutrient Values — Early studies show that radiation can affect the vital essential fatty acids and amino acids in natural foods. In addition, some destruction of vitamins A, B, C, and E will occur. But the FDA says that radiation at the relatively low levels allowed are not a cause for consumer fears. A spokesman for the agency says that the FDA will "look into these concerns further before allowing higher levels."

Critics of the process point out that radiation may destroy the bacteria in foods which cause an unpleasant smell or other obvious signs of spoilage without completely destroying the harmful organisms themselves. This means that we just might end up buying foods that look and smell fresh, but which harbor harmful bacteria.

Consumer groups say that the amount of radioactive materials that will go in and out of just one food irradiation plant (three are projected) every five years will be five times the volume of low-level nuclear wastes produced in the U.S. by *all* sources in 1981, the latest year for which figures are available. Disposing of nuclear power waste is already a serious problem, with many states banning transport across their state boundaries. And we still haven't touched on the dangers to workers, the environment, and the local community in the event of an accident.

Incidentally, the Energy Department is offering waste from nuclear weapons production for the irradiation of foods. That's one way to dispose of 'hot' waste for a profit. First they dump aluminum byproduct wastes (fluoride) in our drinking water (See FLUORIDE this chapter), and now they're using nuclear waste to 'nuke' our foods.

What Can We Do To Protect Ourselves? — Soon the federal government will begin a campaign aimed at persuading America of the 'benefits' and 'safety' of irradiated foods. Don't be fooled. Write to state, local, and U.S. officials of your legitimate concerns. The ultimate protest is simply to refuse to purchase radiated foods. Alert your friends and neighbors to the facts and talk to supermarket owners. If an informed public boycotts 'nuked' foods en masse, the manufacturers and food sellers watching their profit margins drop will get the message in a hurry.

COFFEE & TEA — Along with that caffeine boost you think you need, you are ingesting other substances completely alien to the blood (theobromine, theine, tannin). These toxic elements enter the bloodstream and are carried to the brain, heart, pancreas, spleen, and other organs and glands. The liver and kidneys try valiantly to cleanse and detoxify the contaminated blood and often end up overtired, overworked, and exhausted by their efforts.

If you usually consume a lot of coffee and/or tea, but doubt they are addictive, try eliminating them from your diet abruptly. You'll probably experience withdrawal symptoms ranging from violent headaches to nausea to the shakes. If your health is important to you, it's worth going through the withdrawal period. Science confirms that simply eliminating coffee, and tea (plus cocoa and soda drinks) from the diet can result in a healthy reduction of high blood pressure, reduces the load on the heart, and reopens the arteries supplying the brain.

ANIMAL FATS — For the first time since 1978, the American Heart Association has issued an update on what they call the 'Healthy Heart Dietary Guidelines.' According to Heart Association data, released at a news conference in Washington, D.C.

on August 26, 1986, over half a million Americans will die this year of heart disease. They estimate that upwards of 63 million of us have some form of heart dysfunction and serious blood vessel involvement right now.

The American Heart Association has declared all-out war on the 54 billion dollar per year fast food industry by targeting hamburgers as the number one source of saturated fats in the American diet. According to Association statistics, the hamburger accounts for 20 percent of the saturated fat intake on American menus. The 'Healthy Heart' guidelines call for saturated fats to be limited to a scant 10 percent of our daily calorie count, but current consumption totals between 15 and 20 percent and is viewed as a serious threat to health.

Note: The Heart Association dietary guidelines also say that we should reduce sodium consumption to 2½ grams (one teaspoon) per day. We are also advised to eat more fresh vegetables and fruits, more greens, lean meats and fish, and take only low-fat dairy products. The American Cancer Society is in full agreement with the American Heart Association. Please see Chapter 4 for a complete review of the ACS guidelines.

Without exception, medical authorities everywhere agree that we simply must reduce our consumption of saturated animal fats. If you're a fast-food fanatic and resist giving up your greasy burgers, try these figures on for size. The *Center for Science in the Public Interest* (Washington, D.C.) recently tested and rated the almighty all-American hamburgers produced by some of the more popular burger palaces across the country for saturated fat content. Here's what they found out:

SATURATED FAT CONTENT IN FAST-FOOD HAMBURGERS

- *Carl's Jr.* — The Famous Star Burger
  — 23.6 percent fat
- *Jack in the Box* — The Jumbo Jack
  — 23.4 percent fat
- *Denny's* — regular hamburger
  — 22.3 percent fat

Continued, next page

Continued...

- *Hardee's* — regular hamburger
  - 21.7 percent fat
- *Roy Rogers* — regular hamburger
  - 21.3 percent fat
- *McDonald's* — Quarter Pounder
  - 20.2 percent fat
- *Burger King* — Whopper
  - 20.1 percent fat
- *Wendy's* — regular hamburger
  - 20.6 percent fat
- *D'Lites* — The D'Lite
  - 17.1 percent fat

It appears that we like our hamburgers greasy and full of fat. While we're still on the subject of burgers, a homemade burger (broiled) made with regular ground beef (which is 70 to 75 percent fat before cooking) ends up containing around 19.8 percent fat.

You'll be a little better off if you opt for fast roast beef, but keep in mind you'll still be consuming saturated animal fat. *Arby's* regular roast beef sandwich registered a relatively low 13 percent fat, but is made with processed beef consisting of chunks of untrimmed sirloin and round processed with water, salt, and food-grade phosphates. We are misled into believing we're getting 'roast beef' like mother used to make because the firm then packs the blend into the shape of a roast. *Roy Rogers* roast beef *is* roast beef (top round with the fat trimmed) and came in at only 1.4 percent fat.

Note: After pointing an accusing finger at many of the fast-food chains above, we should add a word of praise here for Denny's. This chain has prepared a series of four brochures about their various food offerings which are available at the cash register, free for the taking.

Here's a quick booklet review: *Dine to your Heart's Content* lists Denny's menu items which are said to follow the American Heart Association guidelines and shows the cholesterol content of each. *Salt Away* helps consumers on low sodium diets choose low-salt foods and shows the content of sodium in many selections. This booklet also informs us that a salt-substitute is available on request. *For Sensitive People* targets foods prepared with MSG (monosodium glutamate), sulfites, and lactose — common food additives that cause an allergic reaction in many. *Waist Not, Want Not* offers a quick review of menu items with 550 calories or less for weight-watchers. It also provides some low-calorie substitution suggestions, such as using lemon and vinegar in place of a high-calorie salad dressing, and touts a low calorie syrup, which is available on request. Three cheers for Denny's for making this important nutritional information readily available to their patrons.

COWS' MILK — As long as we're attacking all the sacred cows that have become so firmly entrenched in our culture, we might as well say a word here about the fat content of the cows' milk we put on the family table as well. We have long been taught that cows' milk is the perfect food, and so it is — for calves. We don't take it directly from the cow herself, of course.

Cows' milk usually comes to us pasteurized, homogenized and frosty cold, very appetizing indeed, especially when served in clear crystal. We urge our children: 'Drink your milk, dear. It makes strong bones and teeth.' However, I remind you that man is the only creature in the world who continues *unnecessarily* to drink milk after being weaned. If you question the truth of that statement, you should know that the enzymes the human body requires to digest milk gradually disappear and are no longer available to the body after age three.

The elements present in both mothers' milk and cows' milk varies according to the diet taken by the donor. The fatty acid content of cows' milk totals about 3.5 percent, with only a very small percentage of the total fat content in the form of the essentials (linoleic and linolenic). But the inner construction of the cow's four stomachs results in a heavy secretion of bacteria which saturates and destroys the value of the essential fatty acids.

The dairy industry could provide the cow with special feed, shown in tests to boost the percentage of usuable essential fats present in the milk, but this especially processed feed is very expensive. Another drawback is that the milk from cows 'fed this type of feed tastes unpleasant and may be doubly harmful. The chemical (formaldehyde) used to process the special feed which kills the bacteria in the cow's stomach that destroys the essential fatty acids is a known carcinogen. But don't waste time worrying about it. This feed is cost prohibitive and will never catch on.

If you think eliminating cows' milk will cause your teeth to rot and your bones to fail from lack of calcium, I have another surprise for you. The calcium present in cows' milk is in a very heavy form, difficult for the human body to process and assimilate efficiently. In addition, this calcium is mixed up with the protein *casein,* which is the principal amino acid in cheeses and milk curds. Both the calcium and casein in cows' milk are easily digested when they pass through the four stomachs of a baby calf, but have a hard time making their way through the human digestive tract. Cows' milk contains 300 times *more* casein than mothers' milk.

You won't have to worry about a calcium deficiency if you are following the dietary recommendations put forth by the medical authorities cited in this book. The good green leafy vegetables, most fruits, and all nuts are rich sources of easily absorbed calcium. Seeds (raw) are excellent sources of calcium. In fact, sesame seeds are delicate, delicious, and extremely high in quality calcium.

AVOIDABLE CARCINOGENS

TOBACCO — No matter how much the tobacco companies may try to make us believe that there is no conclusive evidence linking tobacco use with cancer, is there anyone out there who still goes along with that desperate line of malarky? It can't be long before the Marlboro man falls off his horse and gasps his last. Because of the documented danger to health posed by smoking, and because more and more smokers are giving up their habit, it can be truly said that — in more ways than one — smokers *are* a dying breed. The harmful effects of smoking have been well publicized. Unless you've been deliberately ignoring the onslaught of information, you know that smoking fosters the development of cancer, heart disease, and more.

K.E. Stanley, Ph.D., of the World Health Organization, publishing in *Cancer Detection & Prevention* (Volume 9:83-89, 1986) points out that over one million premature deaths are caused each year by cigarette smoking. Around the world, lung cancer is the second most common form of malignancy (only stomach cancer accounts for more deaths), with close to 600,000 new cases being diagnosed every year. Between 80 and 90 percent of all lung cancer cases are caused by tobacco. The experts say that the risk is greatest among those who start smoking at a young age and among those who smoke strong, unfiltered cigarettes. Dr. Stanley says, "What is needed now is the implementation of national programs of education and legislation with the objective to establish nonsmoking as the cultural norm. There is probably nothing we could do in the way of prevention that would have a larger impact — not only on cancer incidence, but also on cardiovascular diseases and chronic lung diseases — than eliminating tobacco smoking."

Science says that smoking plays a major part in the development of cancer (lung, bladder, esophagus, mouth, throat), emphysema, bronchial problems, and cardiovascular disease. The most hideous aspect of these often deadly conditions is that they take years to develop. Danger signs usually don't appear until the disease is well along and difficult to treat. Early symptoms that smoking is adversely affecting the body include chronic shortness of breath, excessive tiredness, morning headaches, the typical 'smoker's cough,' hoarseness, diminished circulation resulting in a pale complexion, an impaired sense of taste and smell, prematurely aged skin, and sores and/or tenderness of the gums, tongue, and lips. A smoker is intimately acquainted with these symptoms and usually deals with the problems they create by ignoring them.

When a smoker is forced to quit because of serious illness — or gets smart and decides to give up the habit before early problems escalate into an irreversible condition he will experience some withdrawal symptoms, not as severe as those a drug addict suffers, but just as real. Mild discomfort can include a feeling of dizziness, light-headedness, and drowsiness. Anyone with a real desire to quit can handle these minor symptoms. But the nicotine withdrawal symptom that is hardest to overcome (and live with) is a case of screaming nerves. This is the danger point. It's just so easy to light up and feed the habit.

The smokers among us just can't pretend any longer that they're only hurting themselves either. *Second-hand smoke* is the target of the latest research, resulting in some hard legislative action against smokers all across the country — with good reason.

Great-grandmother used to send great-grandfather out behind the barn when he just had to have a smoke so that her horsehair sofa and the heavy velvet drapes in her front parlor wouldn't reek. She had the right idea, but for the wrong reasons. If a loved one (or co-worker) won't stop smoking for his own good health, and many people won't, he should know that he is endangering the health of the entire family. Inhaling second-hand smoke has been documented as a real health hazard. Studies show that non-smokers breathe in as much of the principle cancer-causing compound in smoke (equivalent to smoking four cigarettes) just by spending one hour in the same room with smokers.

The 'sidestream smoke' which exits directly into the atmosphere from the burning tobacco contains twice the amount of tar and nicotine as is in second-hand smoke (which is 'filtered' through the smoker), and between three and five times as much notoriously harmful elements (cadmium, nitrous oxides, benzopyrene, and carbon monoxide), plus a whopping fifty times as much ammonia as is in the smoke that the smoker himself inhales. Children who live with smokers are triply endangered, first, because they are forced to inhale all those harmful substances; second, because their lungs and bodies are small; and third, because studies show they will most likely become smokers themselves.

If you can't quit for yourself, quit for those you love. After all, you wouldn't deliberately infect a loved one with a terminal disease. Why subject them to the harmful effects of second-hand smoke?

HOW TO QUIT — A few years ago, *aversion therapy* (every puff was accompanied by a mild electric shock) enjoyed a brief vogue, but didn't prove successful over the long term. *Medical hypnosis* continues to be popular, but doesn't eliminate the need for will power. Stop-Smoking programs utilizing a form of *group therapy support* are provided by many hospitals and health organizations. These programs report a high success rate. And, a new nicotine-resin impregnated *chewing gum* (Nicorette) is purported to ease nicotine withdrawal symptoms and help conquer the psychological problems associated with quitting smoking. It cannot be taken by a pregnant or nursing mother and must be prescribed by a physician, but it might be worth talking to your doctor about.

Many successful quitters say that going *cold turkey* and simply stopping smoking all at once works better than anything else. If you are truly addicted, remember that after just 72 hours, the worst will be over. By the end of 5 days, the majority find their craving for nicotine is either eliminated, or is so diminished that it is no longer a problem. In contrast, those who have tried *tapering-off* by consciously reducing the number of cigarettes they smoke daily find it more difficult to make that all-important final break.

For a quick detoxification program that works, you should know that studies have shown that megadoses of Vitamin C, when combined with *cysteine* (an amino acid found abundantly in bee pollen, sunflower and sesame seeds) is able to assist the body in detoxifying nicotine. The B vitamins, plus C and cysteine, also fight the harmful effects of *acetaldehyde,* an irritating element present in tobacco smoke. And, no matter how much you *think* you need a smoke, wait 60 seconds. You may be surprised to find that the craving isn't as strong as you thought. When the urge strikes, practice deep breathing. Smokers are usually shallow breathers who only breathe deeply when they inhale.

A national movement backed by the American Cancer Society, the American Heart Association, and the American

Medical Association is aimed at the 30 percent of U.S. adults who are still smokers. You may soon be denied the right to puff away on air flights. A new report by the National Academy of Sciences has determined that the second-hand smoke drifting through the plane from the Smoking Section is harmful to both the crew and non-smoking passengers. Scrapings taken from the air vents shows a heavy concentration of the dangerous pollutants present in tobacco smoke. The problem is compounded because many airlines routinely cut back on the force of their ventilation systems once the plane is off the ground to save fuel, thereby reducing operating costs.

The National Academy of Sciences report has gone to the Transportation Department, accompanied by condemning commentary prepared by the ACS, the AHA, and the AMA. If the legislation is pushed through, smoking may be completely banned on the more than 16,000 domestic flights that cross the country every day. However, the controversy promises to be a lengthy one. The tobacco industry is marshalling its forces, but the medical scientists have a powerful rebuttal ready this time.

SMOKELESS TOBACCO — The practice of dipping snuff and chewing tobacco used to be confined primarily to the rural south. However, for the past few years, tobacco companies have staged a concentrated advertising campaign aimed at our young men. Media ads and television spots featuring sports personalities and entertainers have made a habit which was once considered 'nasty' and 'dirty' into one now thought to be attractive, 'macho,' and less harmful than smoking. Not true.

As a matter of fact, the smokeless tobacco user is at greater risk of developing oral cancer than the smoker. Data developed by the American Cancer Society shows that the risk of developing oral cancer is more than twice as high for the smokeless tobacco addict as for the smoker and that risk increases markedly with long-term exposure. According to statistics from the ACS (Epidemiology & Statistics of Cancer Detection), there were upwards of seven million smokeless tobacco users in the U.S. in 1984 alone. More recent estimates range as high as twenty-two million users, increasing at the terrifying rate of 11 percent every year.

If you or someone you love has been misled into believing that smokeless tobacco is a less harmful form of a proven carcinogen, contact the American Cancer Society and ask for their research reports showing the dangers of smokeless tobacco. ACS has some highly technical material designed to educate health professionals (Cancer Journal for Clinicians), plus some literature (Smokeless Tobacco: Cause for Concern) that is easier reading for the rest of us.

FLUORIDE — *"In point of fact, fluoride causes more human cancer death, and causes it faster, than any other chemical."* So says Dean Burk, Chief Chemist Emeritus of the U.S. National Cancer Institute. As if this statement by a recognized cancer authority isn't damning enough, if you walk into a store to purchase fluoride, it will carry the Skull & Crossbones on its label, the universal symbol for a dangerous poison. In far too many cities across the nation, we are forced to ingest fluoride with our drinking water whether we want to or not. Because this is a free country, we do have several alternatives.

We can go to the expense of purchasing and installing water-purifying equipment that will remove this dangerous carcinogen from our tap water, or we can buy clean water from a delivery service, or we can purchase it by the jug at the store. Of course, we don't like paying several times over for the same product. Not many people can afford to buy clean water for bathing, flushing the commode, and watering the garden, so we have to pay the city water department, *and* we have to pay for drinking and cooking water.

CHEMICALLY-ALTERED FATS — It is an undeniable fact that the incidence of cancer, heart disease, liver and kidney dysfunction, arthritis, multiple sclerosis, and other conditions of fatty degeneration have risen on a parallel course with our consumption of these heavily-advertised dietary fats. There is just too much hard-won evidence that the body cannot process these chemically altered fats. (See Chapter 5.)

Chapter XIII

Getting Back To Basic Nutrition

A Review of the Four Basic Food Groups

Eating right is very simple. All we really need to do is follow the basic *Dietary Guidelines for Americans,* issued in 1980 by the Department of Health & Human Services, as follows:

- Eat a variety of foods
- Maintain ideal weight
- Avoid the wrong kinds of fat
  - chemically-altered fats, saturated animal fats
- Eat foods with adequate complex carbohydrates & fiber
- Avoid sugar and excessive salt

Ever since kindergarten, when colorful pictures of the four basic food groups were commonly posted around the classroom, we have had it drilled into our consciousness that we should eat a measure of each of the four basic food groups every day. Our dietary needs haven't changed over the years. However, what *have* changed are the ways in which foods are manufactured and processed. Dr. Lendon Smith, M.D. said it best: "If man made it, it's probably dangerous." As you review the following chart, be aware that whole foods, not refined and overprocessed foods, are well represented.

260

THE FOUR BASIC FOOD GROUPS

Food Group	Servings Daily	One Serving Equals:
Group #1 Fruits & Vegetables	Four	½ cup juice; ½ cup raw (or cooked) vegetable or fruit; portion commonly served, such as one banana, one medium apple or orange
Group #2 Whole-Grains	Four	1 slice of whole-grain bread; ½ cup cooked whole-grain cereal, rice, pasta, grits; 1 cup of whole-grain ready-to-eat cereal
Group #3 Dairy Products	Two	1 cup of milk (low-fat, or skim); 1 cup yogurt (low-fat, unsugared); 2 cups cottage cheese (low-fat); 1½ ounces cheese (natural, unprocessed)
Group #4 Protein Sources	Two	2 ounces fish, poultry, lean meat; Protein Sources ½ cup cottage cheese (low-fat); 2 eggs; 2 ounces hard cheese; ½ cup dried legumes, peas, beans (cooked)

FRUITS & VEGETABLES — Food Group 1

We should eat four or more servings of fruits and vegetables every day. Most authorities recommend that we eat some fresh fruit daily and a dark green or deep yellow vegetable at least every other day. Because some of the important vitamins are lost in cooking, plan to eat at least a portion of your vegetables (and leafy greens) raw, perhaps in a salad. Along with their healthy content of complex carbohydrates and cleansing fiber, fruits and vegetables supply vitamins A, C, and P (the bioflavonoids).

VITAMIN A — This vital fat-soluble vitamin is manufactured in the body from beta-carotene. It is essential for normal growth and development, for maintainenance of the skin (the largest eliminative organ of the body), and for good teeth and bones. A deficiency of vitamin A lowers our resistance to infections, interferes with our ability to adapt to darkness (night blindness), and can affect the cornea of the eye. Healthy hair growth depends on a sufficient supply of vitamin A as well.

The Institute of Cancer Research at Vienna University (Austria) has reported on approximately 1,150 cancer patients treated with megadoses of vitamin A. This vitamin therapy was shown to enhance the effects of radiation and chemotherapy. Even when vitamin A was used alone against squamous cell carcinomas of the skin, the scientists said that a complete remission was obtained. In a series of experiments with lab animals, vitamin A injections (fortified with amygdalin [see Chapter 12] and natural enzymes) brought dramatic results against massive tumors. After four days of intramuscular injections, a pimple appeared at the site of the tumor. Two days later, the pimple broke open and discharged pus. A microscopic examination of the discharge showed the presence of dead tumor cells. As the pus continued to discharge over time, the tumors receded. Four to six weeks later, over 90 percent of the animals were completely free of tumors.

Note: Because megadoses of vitamin A can result in liver dysfunction, a specially prepared water-soluble form of the vitamin was used in the studies reviewed above. High doses of vitamin A cannot be considered a home treatment.

The University of Arizona (Tucson, Arizona) has published research by F.L. Meyskens, Jr., M.D. showing that applying vitamin A to precancerous cells in the cervix of 18 female patients resulted in six cases of remission after just four days of treatment. And scientists at the Albert Einstein College of Medicine (New York) discovered that women showing evidence of early precancerous changes of the cervix commonly ate a diet deficient in beta-carotene, vitamin A, and vitamin C.

Food Sources of Vitamin A — The green and yellow-orange vegetables are rich sources of natural vitamin A, as are many fruits (prunes, pineapples, oranges, limes, and cantaloupes). Other sources of vitamin A include liver, cod liver oil, butter, milk, and egg yolks.

VITAMIN C — Ascorbic acid (vitamin C) is essential for the formation of connective tissue all over the body. It is the inter-cellular 'glue' which maintains the strength of tissues and cells and is vital for strong capillary walls. Evidence suggests that supplying the body with vitamin C in quantity can protect against the common cold. The *Journal of Human Nutrition* (February 1981) tells us that vitamin C can increase the level of high-density lipoproteins (HDL) in the blood. HDL protects against cardiovascular disease. Nobel prize winner Linus Pauling has documented the fact that cancer patients usually exhibit a very low level of ascorbic acid in their infection-fighting white blood cells (leucocytes). Dr. Pauling has also confirmed that cancer patients given high doses of vitamin C live longer and feel better. Statistics show that a diet high in fruits and vegetables can lower the incidence of stomach cancer.

Food Sources of Vitamin C — The citrus fruits are prime sources of vitamin C, but other fruits (strawberries, apples, pears, apricots, plums, peaches, pineapples) are also good. Many vegetables (rutabagas, tomatoes, onions, carrots, green peppers, radishes, carrots, celery, lettuce) offer a healthy content of vitamin C also.

263

VITAMIN P — The bioflavonoids (rutin, hesperidin, citrin) have been collectively dubbed vitamin P, because they exercise a strengthening effect on the permeability of the capillaries, the tiniest blood vessels. Bioflavonoids are essential for the efficient absorption and assimilation of vitamin C. They also work with vitamin C to keep collagen healthy. Collagen represents about 30 percent of the total protein content of the body. It is an important element of cellular connective tissue, promotes youthful elasticity of the skin, and is a vital part of ligaments, cartilage, and bone.

Food Sources of Vitamin P — Fresh fruits and vegetables are good sources of the bioflavonoids, but they are missing in juices and are largely destroyed by cooking. It is the pulpy part (in vegetables and fruits) and thin skin separating the sections in citrus that provides the Vitamin P. Mother Nature always provides vitamin C and vitamin P in the same foods, because each activates the other. Together, they are more potent and powerful than either is alone. (See *Food Sources of Vitamin C* above.)

COMPLEX CARBOHYDRATES — The complex carbohydrates in fruits and vegetables fill you up, but not out. For years, dieters have considered carbohydrate as the villain in a weight-loss regimen, but complex carbos should actually total more than half of the total calories we eat every day. Carbohydrates are the natural fuel (energy) source of the body, but they serve another important function as well. The body converts complex carbohydrates into energy (glycogen) for short-term storage in the liver. This nutrient protects against toxins and controls the breakdown of proteins. Protein can be used for energy production when necessary, but is absolutely vital for cell growth and repair. By supplying the body with complex carbos, we are protected against the nitrogenous waste that is a by-product of the breakdown of proteins.

Food Sources of Complex Carbohydrates — Nature packs complex carbohydrates into just about everything that grows.

In other words, all foods of plant origin are high in the complex carbohydrates essential to life. Remember, it's the *refined* carbohydrates and empty calories present in over-processed manufactured food items that contribute to obesity and many other health problems, not nature's pure version of this important nutrient.

FIBER — The recommendation of the American Cancer Society that we increase our intake of fiber is based on solid research showing that societies which commonly consume a diet high in fiber have a very low incidence of colorectal and intestinal cancers. The difference between these so-called primitive civilizations and our highly industrialized country is primarily one of bowel habits. African natives, for instance, may empty their bowels as often as two or three times every day.

Close to 15 percent of all cancer deaths in this country in 1982, according to the National Cancer Institute (Surveillance, Epidemiology & End Results), were caused by colon and rectal cancers. The body is designed to excrete waste after every meal, but we have come to believe that it's 'normal' to have a bowel movement twice a week. Constipation is a national problem. But certain elements in bile acids can turn into cancer-causing carcinogens. When these carcinogenic substances stay in contact with the colon for a lengthy period, such as when we are constipated, a malignancy can develop. The experts say that simply increasing our intake of fiber, thereby eliminating the constipation factor, can reduce this frightening statistic markedly.

Another factor in favor of fiber is that it is a good source of *silicon*. Silicon occurs in the skeletal structure and teeth, helps maintain the integrity of the arterial system, and assists in strengthening connective tissue all over the body. The experts believe silicon is a preventive against heart disease and arthritis.

Food Sources of Fiber — Of the fruits and vegetables, the best sources of fiber are fresh blackberries, fresh apples, dried figs, dried dates, broccoli, cauliflower, parsnips, pumpkin, and rutabaga. There is another very good source of fiber. See below.

WHOLE GRAINS (BREADS, CEREALS) —
Food Group 2

A healthy diet should include four or more servings of whole grain foods every day. Grains are truly the staff of life for most of the world. In the Far East, rice is eaten at every meal. In the Middle East, the cuisine features bulgur (parboiled wheat). We all know (and love) the pasta of Italy. In the Soviet bloc countries, black bread is a delicious and healthy staple. And many of us have become acquainted with the tortillas that are the backbone of the menu south-of-the-border.

But, in America (sometimes called the 'breadbasket of the world'), we often bypass the staff of life. We just don't have a favorite grain that we serve with every meal. Oh, sure, we may give the children a bowl of cereal before sending them off to school. But very often we are serving the 'latest' in a long string of artificially colored 'cereals' (which tint the milk with dye) made popular by colorful (and repetitive) kid-oriented TV commercials. This cereal is probably also over-refined, heavily sugared, and contains many additives.

Whole grain products provide complex carbohydrates, B and E vitamins, iron, magnesium (and traces of other minerals), and more of the healthy fiber we need. The protein in whole grains is incomplete. On a completely vegetarian diet, plant proteins are made complete by eating foods containing the missing amino acids (legumes, milk) at the same meal.

THE B COMPLEX VITAMINS — The water-soluble vitamins known collectively as B Complex include: thiamine (B1), riboflavin (B2), niacin (B3, or nicotinic acid), pyridoxine (B6), biotin, inositol, p-aminobenzoic acid (PABA), cyanocobalamine (B12), pantothenic acid, and folic acid. Medical science has determined that a lack of any one of the Bs brings on a host of medical problems. In other words, we need them all.

The B vitamins affect the growth processes, appetite, the gastro-intestinal tract, the nervous system, the endocrine glands (especially the adrenals), reduce blood sugar levels in diabetes, are necessary for carbohydrate metabolism, and are useful in treating tuberculosis. To give you a grasp of just how important the entire complex of Bs are, consider: A deficiency of B complex can result in an enlarged liver, degeneration of the sex glands, an upset of the nervous system, and can cause a dysfunction of the heart, liver, spleen, kidneys, pituitary, salivary, and adrenal glands.

Food Sources of B Complex — The primary source of the B vitamins are the whole grains and unpolished brown rice. Other sources of one or more of the Bs include Brewer's yeast, legumes, nuts, green vegetables, poultry, eggs, fruits, fish, and meats (pork, liver, beef, and veal). However, it would be unwise in the extreme to use a diet high in meats to get your B complex at the expense of the whole grains. The unhealthy content of saturated fats in meats make them a suspect addition to the menu.

VITAMIN E — Medical science acknowledges that vitamin E is an essential nutrient for man. Over the past decade, many researchers have been studying the action of this antioxidant, known to protect against the harmful development of certain elements which destroy cells. Science has determined that sufficient vitamin E protects against cardiovascular disease (coronary thrombosis, rheumatic heart disease, angina, hypertensive heart disease), phlebitis, supports the immune system, and reduces cramping (menstrual, night cramps, during exercise). Because vitamin E is known to support the immune system, many health authorities believe it is a good addition to the anti-cancer diet as well.

Food Sources of Vitamin E — Good natural sources of dietary vitamin E include wheat germ, whole grains, and soybeans. Additional sources are beans, some fruits and vegetables, and liver. Note: To protect the essential fatty acids (linoleic and linolenic) from oxidation, vitamin E (as a primary natural antioxidant) has been documented as a necessary adjunct to a diet high in polyunsaturates.

IRON — Because iron is essential to the formation of healthy red blood cells (hemoglobin), it is essential to life. Iron is absorbed from food in the small intestines and is transported, via the bloodstream, to bone marrow, where the production of red blood cells is accomplished. As a component of hemoglobin, iron is essential for the transport of oxygen needed for tissue respiration. A lack of iron leads to anemia, retarded development, and low vitality. Iron deficient individuals very often have an abnormally pale complexion.

Food Sources of Iron — Whole wheat, bran, graham, and oatmeal are all excellent sources of iron. Other good sources include almonds, eggs, oysters, soy beans, liver, kidney, many fruits (apricots, currants, dates, oranges, prunes, raisins, rhubarb), and a lot of vegetables (asparagus, beans, cauliflower, celery, chard, dandelions, lettuce, beets, cabbage, cucumbers, parsnips, peppers, peas, potatoes, radishes, tomatoes, turnips, mushrooms).

However, only a fraction of the organic iron present in foods is absorbed by the body. Medical science says that it's necessary to provide from 15 to 30 mg of iron in the diet to be sure that from 1.0 to 4.0 mg will be absorbed.

MAGNESIUM — The healthy human body contains approximately 25 gm of magnesium, most of which is in the bones. Even a small increase in dietary magnesium has been shown to markedly increase bone density. But this white mineral element is also present in the cells, soft tissues, muscles, and in the body fluids. Magnesium is required to activate important enzymes and is associated with the regulation of body temperature, neuromuscular contractions, the metabolism of fats, and the synthesis of proteins. A concentration of this important nutrient (second only to potassium) is found in all cells.

It has been noted that the spinal fluid of hibernating animals contains a high amount of magnesium. It is believed that muscle tremors (and possibly a tendency to convulsions) may be controlled by adding magnesium to the diet. As one of nature's relaxing nutrients, magnesium taken at bedtime promotes healthy sleep. A lack of magnesium can result in erratic or rapid heart beat (implicated in myocardial infarction), low blood pressure, fatigue, mood swings, depression, anxiety, calcium deposits, kidney stones, and even dental problems. Studies show that laboratory animals given feed with less than two parts per million of magnesium sicken and die.

Food Sources of Magnesium — The experts tell us that magnesium is obtained in sufficient quantity in our daily meals — just as long as the menu includes a good measure of the whole grains, fresh fruits, and fresh vegetables. Excellent sources of magnesium include beans, seeds (pumpkin, sesame, sunflower), almonds, and soybeans.

MANGANESE — Manganese is an essential element needed for normal bone development, and it participates in many enzyme reactions as well. It is involved in fat metabolism and protein synthesis, and assists the cells in the production of energy.

A deficiency of manganese is often exhibited by diabetics, epileptics, and myasthenia gravis victims. A lack of this mineral is believed to contribute to some back problems, sterility, dizziness, tinnitus (noises within the ear), lack of coordination, and apathy. As an aid to the diabetic, supplemental manganese can improve glucose tolerance. Because manganese stimulates important neurotransmitters in the brain, it has been demonstrated to improve memory in some cases. Researchers have discovered that male laboratory animals deprived of manganese become sterile; females deprived of manganese lack the maternal instinct and will not care for their young.

Food Sources of Manganese — The whole grains (bran included) are excellent sources of dietary manganese. Additional sources include seeds, nuts, eggs, legumes, the green leafy vegetables, and blueberries.

MOLYBDENUM — An interesting natural phenomenon is that organic foods which offer vitamin C must have molybdenum in order to produce vitamin C. Molybdenum is required to activate certain enzymes. It is an essential trace element in plant growth, where it is used as a catalyst in fixing nitrogeneous proteins. New Zealand researchers have determined that, as an important trace mineral, molybdenum can protect against tooth decay.

Food Sources of Molybdenum — The whole grains offer molybdenum, as do legumes and green leafy vegetables.

POTASSIUM — Potassium is the principal element in intracellular fluid and is of primary importance. A proper balance of potassium, calcium, and magnesium is required for normal heart action and for the conduction of nerve impulses. A potassium deficiency results in a heart dysfunction, marked weakness of the muscles, dizziness, thirst, and mental confusion.

Food Sources of Potassium — Potassium is present in varying levels in many foods, but the best sources of dietary potassium include the cereal grains, dried peas, and dried beans. Additional sources include fresh vegetables, fresh fruits, fresh fish, fresh poultry, nuts, and molasses.

DAIRY PRODUCTS — Food Group 3

Milk contains a generous amount of protein (see Food Group 4) and calcium, plus the vitamins A, B2, B6, and B12 (see Food Group 2), and is usually fortified with vitamin D. Daily requirements as set forth in the government guidelines say: Adults should take 2 cups of milk; children up to 9 years should take 2 to 3 cups; children 9 to 12 (and pregnant women) should take 3 to 4 cups; young adults 12 to 18 (and nursing mothers) should take 4 cups or more. In all the above daily recommendations, the equivalent in milk products may be substituted for all or a portion of the milk. (See Chapter 12 for some drawbacks to the consumption of cows' milk.)

Food Sources of Dairy Products — Other popular dairy products which may be used in place of milk include cottage cheese, yogurt, various cheeses, and even ice cream or ice milk. However, many of these foods are processed with excessive sugar (or artificial sweeteners), chemical additives, and artificial colors (dyes). Please remember to select low-fat dairy products and watch out for the additives.

CALCIUM — Calcium promotes strong teeth and bones, is essential for the functions of the heart, nerves, and muscles, and is also of great importance in regulating the coagulation factor of blood. Calcium is carried in the bloodstream, but unless its companion nutrients (phosphorus, vitamin D) are available in sufficient supply, calcium absorption will not take place.

A deficiency of calcium causes muscle twitching, spasms, and may result in convulsions. It is important to remember that a high fiber diet acts to decrease the body's ability to assimilate calcium and phosphorus (See Food Group 4). This does not mean that we should reduce fiber, but rather we should compensate accordingly by including additional calcium-rich foods in planning daily meals.

Food Sources of Calcium — Milk has come to be accepted as a primary source of dietary calcium, but even better sources include beans, cauliflower, chard, cheese, eggs, kale, molasses, and rhubarb. Science says that a good supply of calcium can be obtained from almonds, beets, bran, cabbage, carrots, celery, dates, figs, kohlrabi, lemons, lettuce, oatmeal, oranges, oysters, parsnips, pineapple, raspberries, rutabagas, shellfish, spinach, turnips, walnuts, and watercress.

VITAMIN D — Because vitamin D is essential in the metabolism of calcium and phosphorus, it is essential for the normal development and maintenance of the skeletal structure and teeth. D is sometimes called the 'sunshine vitamin' because exposure to the sun (or ultraviolet light) synthesizes vitamin D in the body. Without vitamin D, the bones grow soft and/or diseased, rickets develops, and teeth cannot be efficiently remineralized.

Food Sources of Vitamin D — Vitamin D is present in milk (if it has been so enriched), butter, eggs, and fish oils (primarily cod and salmon).

THE PROTEIN SOURCES — Food Group 4

A complete protein is one that contains all the essential amino acids (tryptophane, lysine, methionine, valine, leucine, isoleucine, phenylalanine, threonine, arginine, histidine). Complete protein is essential for growth, the building of new tissue, and the repair of injured or weak tissue. Proteins are used first in the manufacture of red blood cells (hemoglobin), second for the production of blood plasma proteins, and third in tissue repair where needed. Proteins form an integral part of the protoplasm of every cell in the body and are essential to the life processes.

Food Sources of Protein — Because we are traditionally a meat-eating society, the first protein source which springs to mind is meat, especially red meat. However, we must keep the strong recommendation of both the American Cancer Society and the American Heart Association that we reduce our consumption of saturated animal fats firmly in mind when considering the food sources of proteins.

Fish, poultry, eggs, and bee pollen are all excellent sources of rich protein, as are the legumes (beans, peas, lentils, chickpeas), seeds, and nuts. Yes, peanuts are a good source of protein. But commercially processed peanut butters are both sugared and made with partially hydrogenated oils. (See Chapter 5.) Health food stores offer a natural version containing nothing but ground peanuts. Because natural peanut butters are not homogenized, the peanut oil will rise to the top. If you want a peanut butter that comes close to the commercial varieties, you may want to blend in a little honey and a pinch of salt.

COPPER — Copper mates with iron in the manufacture of red blood cells, but about three-quarters of the body's copper is in the bones. Some authorities believe a deficiency of copper is implicated in the development of osteoporosis. It makes a vital contribution to the skeletal structure and helps maintain the integrity of the arterial system. Because so many homes are fitted with copper plumbing, an excess of copper is more common than a deficiency.

Food Sources of Copper — In nature, copper sources include liver, nuts, and oysters.

LECITHIN — Lecithin is one of the 'friendly fats,' shown in research to help hold harmful cholesterol in suspension in the bloodstream, thereby preventing the buildup of the atherosclerotic plaque implicated in heart disease. Lecithin also offers choline (an important amino acid) and steps up the body's production of acetylcholine (a neurotransmitter). Autopsies confirm that acetylcholine is notably low in the brains of Alzheimer's disease victims. The prestigious British medical journal *Lancet* has reported that individuals with Alzheimer's disease (and some forms of learning disabilities) can be helped by adding lecithin to the diet.

Food Sources of Lecithin — The highest concentration of lecithin in nature is found in the yolk of eggs, debunking the medical admonition of some years ago that eating eggs contributes to high cholesterol levels.

PHOSPHORUS — This is another mineral important to the strength and density of bones and teeth, essential in the absorption and utilization of calcium. Phosphorus compounds are the principal sources of energy in muscle contractions, and its presence is required to enable the body to convert glycogen to glucose, our prime source of energy.

Food Sources of Phosphorus — Phosphorus is found in the proteins of food. Excellent sources of phosphorus include almonds, beans, barley, bran, cheese, eggs, lentils, liver, milk, oatmeal, peanuts, peas, walnuts, whole wheat, and rye.

SULFUR — Sulfur is an important element present in every cell of both animals and plants. It is required for the synthesis of proteins and collagen. A deficiency affects the skin and nails, and contributes to both anemia and hair loss. Sulfur works with the B complex vitamins and assists in the efficient metabolism of the essential fatty acids.

Food Sources of Sulfur — Cottage cheese (low-fat) is a primary source of the sulfur-rich proteins (recommended in conjunction with linseed oil [see Chapter 6] by Dr. Johanna Budwig). Many other foods contain sulfur, including eggs, peanuts, onions, garlic, and whole cereal grains.

ZINC — The breast milk of a new nursing mother contains a strong concentration of zinc for the first two weeks, with a sharp drop noted after that period. A newborn child's liver contains three times as much zinc as the liver of an adult, showing that nature considers this mineral vital for normal development. Zinc is always present in human tissues, but the greatest concentration occurs in the thyroid and sex organs at adulthood. Zinc contributes to a wide variety of bodily functions, but requires the help of vitamin A. It is vitamin A which mates with zinc stored in the liver. Zinc and vitamin A are commonly given together for the treatment of acne, eczema, and psoriasis.

A study conducted at Purdue University (Lafayette, Indiana) determined that close to 60 percent of adult Americans over the age of 60 lack zinc. Early symptoms of a zinc deficiency include a measurable loss of taste and smell, and wounds that heal poorly and slowly. Other research has shown that the blood of rheumatoid arthritis victims is markedly lacking in zinc. When zinc was replaced in the diet, the arthritic patients reported less early morning stiffness, less swelling of joints, and found they could walk for a longer period of time without pain. Health authorities say that a severe zinc deficiency contributes to cancer, cystic fibrosis, low sperm count in males, prostatitis, a loss of libido, menstrual problems in the female, and toxemia during pregnancy. In medically prescribed doses of 100 mg daily, zinc has been shown to increase the production of antibodies.

Food Sources of Zinc — The natural zinc in foods is almost completely destroyed in commercial food processing. To add to the problem, the zinc content of the soil in most agricultural states has been exhausted. The experts say that a good diet should include approximately 15 mg of zinc daily. The best sources are liver (3 ounces yields 6 mg of zinc), and peanut butter (3 ounces yields 3 mg of zinc).

WHAT'S MISSING FROM THE FOUR BASIC FOOD GROUPS?

ESSENTIAL FATTY ACIDS — There is a vast quantity of material in this book showing the important functions of the essential fatty acids (linoleic and linolenic). Remember, 'essential' means just that. The body cannot manufacture linoleic or linolenic fatty acids from other elements. They must be supplied daily in the diet. (See Chapters 5 & 6.)

Food Sources of the Essential Fatty Acids — There has been quite a bit written lately about the benefits of olive oil and salmon oil. While both are good sources of fatty acids, neither one contains both linoleic and linolenic fatty acids. The best sources of the essential fatty acids in human nutrition are linseed oil, soybean oil, pumpkin oil, and walnut oil. Only these four oils, and *only when they are not altered in processing,* offer both essential fatty acids. Please see chart below.

ESSENTIAL FATTY ACIDS CONTENT OF COMMON VEGETABLE OILS

Source	Fat Content Total %	Essential Fatty Acids Linolenic	Linoleic	Both Essentials Total %
Linseed	35	58	14	72
Soybean	18	9	50	59
Pumpkin	47	15	42	57
Walnut	60	5	51	56
Rapeseed*	30	7	30	37
Safflower	59	0	75	
Sunflower	47	0	65	
Grape	Trace	0	71	
Corn	4	0	59	
Wheat Germ	10	0	54	
Sesame	49	0	54	
Rice Bran	10	0	35	
Cotton**	Trace	0	50	
Peanut***	47	0	29	
Almond	54	0	17	
Macadamia	71	0	10	
Cashew	41	0	6	
Olive	20	0	8	
Coconut	35	0	3	
Palm Kernel	35	0	3	

* Rapeseed (canola) contains toxic *erucic acid*

** Cottonseed contains common toxins

*** Peanuts (damp) harbor a toxic fungus

Hemp (not listed because it is illegal in the U.S.) provides both essential fatty acids

SELENIUM — This powerful antioxidant has been shown in scientific research to inhibit the formation of tumors, probably by stimulating the production of important antibodies. Lab animals first given selenium and then deliberately exposed to toxic chemicals were found to have developed a degree of immunity to the toxins. The National Cancer Institute has said that just 200 mcg (micrograms) of selenium daily might be a cancer preventive. Based on on-going animal and human studies, the experts are saying that cancer rates across the board could be decreased over the long term by as much as 70 percent if the general population merely ingested this small of amount of selenium daily. Japanese women, who commonly consume a diet which provides from 250 to 350 mcg of selenium daily, have a very low rate of breast cancer, just one-fifth that of American women.

Food Sources of Selenium — Natural dietary selenium has become difficult to find. As long ago as 1965, studies showed conclusively that persons living in areas where selenium was present in strong concentration in the soil and water enjoyed a lower rate of cancer than the national average. Unfortunately, some chemical fertilizers (sulfates) inhibit selenium development in food crops, and the soil in a vast number of states is deficient (or totally devoid) of selenium.

Foods grown in North Dakota, South Dakota, and/or Nebraska still offer a good content of natural selenium. If you live in these states and/or eat foods grown in these states, you're in luck. For the rest of us an alternative to consider is a comprehensive blend of bee pollens harvested in the Dakotas and other western states because they provide a healthy amount of natural selenium, and other very important healthy nutrients.

NUTRITION AND HEALTH

If you're still not convinced that what we eat controls how we feel and the degree of health we enjoy, here's what some medical scientists and recognized health authorities have found.

Kanematsu Sugiura, M.D., a researcher at the Sloan-Kettering Cancer Institute, discovered a few years ago that *amygdalin,* a natural substance found in many seeds and nuts, better known as laetrile or B17 (see Chapter 12) is a powerful inhibitor of cancer. Dr. Sugiura's report states, "Amygdalin caused regression (of tumors) in 80 percent of the animals studied, and complete regression in 40 percent. There is a significant inhibition of the formation of lung metastases and it possibly prevents, to an uncertain degree, the formation of new tumors." Sloan-Kettering suppressed Dr. Sugiura's report and discontinued research on the properties of amygdalin.

Another nutrient source which showed great promise in early testing as a natural cancer inhibitor was bee pollen. (See Chapter 8.) U.S. government studies (Department of Agriculture) investigating the benefits of bee pollen were dropped with no explanation.

Important research conducted by A.B. Robinson, Ph.D. at the Linus Pauling Institute (Menlo Park, California) shows conclusively the part diet plays in conquering cancer. After inducing cancer in laboratory animals, Group 1 was given a diet consisting only of apples, bananas, carrots, pears, sunflower seeds, tomatoes and wheat grass. Group 2 was given very high vitamin C (along with commercially manufactured feed). Group 3 was given high vitamin C in addition to the same raw diet fed to Group 1. The results were definitive. In the animals in Group 1 and Group 2, the cancerous lesions were reduced five-fold. But in Group 3, given both the raw diet *and* high vitamin C, an astounding and very satisfying 35-times decrease in cancerous lesions was achieved. Dr. Robinson points out, "The incidence of severe cancerous lesions in these experiments was caused to vary over a 70-fold range by *nutritional measures alone."*

Albert Schweitzer, physician, humanitarian, and winner of the Nobel Peace Prize in 1952, was astounded to discover a completely cancer-free society on his arrival in French Equatorial Africa in 1913. Dr. Schweitzer wrote: "I was astonished to encounter no cases of cancer. I saw none among the natives 200 miles from the coast. This absence of cancer seems to be due to the difference in *nutrition of the natives,* as compared to the Europeans."

From 1942 to 1946, a steady decrease in the number of dental caries (cavities) was documented in the population of Norway. The reason? Food rationing during World War II took sugar and other refined carbohydrates off the market. In place of refined over-processed foods, Norwegians were taking vegetables, bread, potatoes, and milk. By 1947, the eating of refined foods had returned to pre-war levels and the incidence of dental problems kept pace.

As long ago as 1944, an article by Dr. H.H. Turner published in the *Pennsylvania Medical Journal* pointed out that close to 90 percent of the adults over age 45 had vision problems. Dr. Turner expressed his belief that the carbonic acid found in carbonated soft-drinks (sodas), devoured in large quantities by a huge percentage of the population, was responsible for the great increase in near-sightedness (myopia) in the U.S.

"America is one of the sickest and worst fed nations on earth." So states J.C. Nichols, M.D., a noted medical writer. Dr. R.J. Williams, professor of biochemistry, the University of Texas (Austin, Texas), states without equivocation, "Enumerating various changes characteristic of aging (impaired vision, hearing, memory, strength and endurance decline, insomnia, loss of libido and appetite for food, aches and pains, increased tendency toward constipation, arthritis, diabetes, arteriosclerosis, osteoporosis, senility, etc.), I want to call attention to the idea that every one of the cells and tissues in the body have to perform their functions properly and also that every one of these failures is related to *cell and tissue nutrition*. We can state with assurance that the longer cells are furnished with the necessities of life, including good nutrition, the longer they will continue to remain in good working order."

The dietary recommendations of the American Cancer Society (and the American Heart Association), reviewed and thoroughly explained in this book, have refined the basic guidelines given above even further. The Director of the National Cancer Institute's prevention program, Dr. Peter Greenwald, has been quoted as saying, "Laboratory studies suggest certain vitamins have an inhibitory effect on cancer."

We remind you that cells and the products of cells form all the tissues of the body. All functions of the body are carried on by cells, both individually and collectively. Cells arise only from preexisting cells by a process of cell division. Growth and development occur from an increase in the numbers of cells and the differentiation of cells into different types of tissues. It is obvious that if we keep the cells in good working order by supplying them with the nutrients they require to proceed with the life processes, we are then practicing a very effective form of preventive medicine indeed.

DEFEATING CANCER

The best cure for cancer is avoiding it altogether. Prevention is the first defense - as you've likely learned from the previous chapters of this book. Other important elements, including basic nutrition, choosing and communicating with a doctor, and using common-sense health practices, are outlined here, as well as some additional alternative treatments for those who've contracted the disease.

Cancer is the most feared of all diseases, but it's not necessarily a death sentence. Many kinds of cancer can be prevented with proper diet and lifestyle. Today's "average diet" creates significant risks for cancer development. The American diet is frequently so poor that the Senate Select Committee on Nutrition and Human Needs studied it and found our diets contain:

Too much food, altogether; we eat too much
Too much red meat
Too much fat
Too much cholesterol
Too much sugar
Too much salt

Recommendations included:

Reduce fat intake to 30 percent of your daily diet
Reduce sugar to 15 percent of your daily diet
Drastically cut salt intake

Studies show that diet and nutrition are factors in 60 percent of cancers in women and 40 percent of cancers in men.

But some of the risk factors are within our control. Eliminating ten of these major risk factors can significantly improve your chances of survival.

FIGHTING CANCER TO WIN: WHAT YOU CAN DO TO AVOID RISKS

1. Maintain your ideal weight; avoid obesity
2. Follow a diet plan modelled after the Food Pyramid
3. Avoid all forms of tobacco; limit alcohol
4. Avoid radiation, sunburn and environmental hazards
5. Avoid drugs, hormones, steroids and unsafe sex practices
6. Avoid refined sugar and sugar substitutes
7. Learn the seven cancer warning signs
8. Know your body and medical history
9. Exercise, avoid stress and have regular medical exams
10. Take a vitamin supplement each day

It seems every time we switch on the news or pick up a paper, some new study has proved another common food or environmental element causes cancer. It seems we cannot count on our federal regulators to keep us safe from cancer risks. We must be informed.

A degree of aggression is important. Be aggressive at seeking out *organically grown produce* and stores that sell it. Find out where and when local farmers market their produce. Look beyond your kitchen table to the legislature and medical fields, which regulate and provide alternative cancer treatments and nutritional supplements.

One example of "nutritional activism" is the Dietary Supplement Health and Information Act, a bill recently introduced to the U.S. Senate. It is designed to give consumers more freedom to information and supplies on herbs, vitamins and other "cures" now consigned to obscurity.

Sen. Orrin Hatch of Utah said he was disgusted at the FDA's restrictions on vitamin supplements and natural cures. "Cancer Chronicals" journal said Hatch told FDA officials "I am dismayed that you want to restrict a citizen's ability to know more about vitamins."

The agency now restricts labeling and access to many types of food supplements, purportedly in an effort to prevent citizens from harming themselves. If passed, the new regulations would allow manufacturers to label their products with dosages and the healthy effects they are supposed to provide. Manufacturers would have to meet strict quality standards while consumers would be given free choice in their self-treatment.

For now, the Nutritional Health Alliance keeps a toll-free information hotline for those interested in vitamin and herbal supplement information. Those with specific questions on vitamins and their uses can call 1-800-226-4NHA.

Other health activists focus on ecology - the wise stewardship of the soil, plants and environment we all depend on for life. This can be achieved in a small way by patronizing farmers and manufacturers who use safe, non-toxic growing and handling methods. Others boycott or write letters to manufacturers who pollute air and water.

But for those more interested in cancer, its treatment and prevention, the following groups provide excellent resources.

National Cancer Institute
Office of Communications
Building 31, Room 10A24
Bethesda, MD 20892
Phone 1-800-4-CANCER.

People Against Cancer:
"The Cancer Chronicles" newsletter
P.O. Box 10
Otho, IA 50569
Phone 1-515-972-4444

This is a non-profit cancer support group.

The FDA "Consumer"
Journal of the Food and Drug Administration
500 Fishers Lane
Rockville, MD 20857
Phone 310-443-9057

"The Consumer" contains articles on nutrition, food additives, current research and breakthroughs.

The People's Medical Society
462 Walnut St.
Allentown, PA 18102
Phone 215-770-1670

This non-profit group publishes "Cancer Care," a newsletter featuring cancer treatments, self-help, and tips on dealing with doctors.

FINDING THE RIGHT DOCTOR

Finding the right doctor is the first step in getting the best healthcare and cancer treatment. Dr. Vincent DeVita, former director of the National Cancer Institute advises patients to always seek a second opinion.

"I've never met a doctor under treatment who didn't get a second opinion, and who didn't get the (laboratory) slides read by two different pathologists." As physician-in-chief at Memorial Sloan-Kettering Cancer Center, DeVita has the authority to say so.

Patients can get referrals from the government's Second Surgical Opinion Hotline: 1-800-638-6833.

When choosing a doctor, look for the following:

The doctor's *interest and thoroughness* in periodic physical exams. If you need special tests, you'll want a doctor who is willing to order them.

The doctor's *ability to listen* when you talk, and his openness to your questions. Don't be afraid to ask a doctor for his qualifications, or if he's treated this type of cancer before. If you don't understand his explanation, ask him to clarify. Remember - you are the one paying the bill.

The doctor's *commitment* to your best interest. If you are sick and require treatment, the doctor should explain all the treatment alternatives available. A good doctor will show you your options, and then allow you to choose. If he rules out particular treatments, you deserve an explanation. He should suggest preventive measures, nutrition and lifestyle changes - not just drugs.

The doctor's *willingness to work with other doctors*. He may need to consult with someone else during your treatment, to ensure you get the best treatment. Avoid a doctor with competitive doctor-vs.-doctor ego mentality.

The doctor's *willingness to stop treatments that aren't working* and *consider other options*. Remember, you are not locked into a treatment that seems to be going nowhere. A good doctor will consider your perspectives on the effectiveness of treatments - but it's important you understand just what your doctor considers "effective."

The doctor's *People Skills*. Do you and your doctor see eye-to-eye? How does he view alternative cancer treatments? Dr. Robert Mayer of the Dana-Farber Cancer Institute wrote in the Harvard Medical School Health Letter that "in most cases, what is needed is not some sort of exotic, high-tech treatment, but the guidance of an organized, sensitive, caring primary physician. Rather than searching for the most overworked specialist they can find, many patients and families would do better to seek a doctor who relates well to patient, who will act as an advocate, and who can undertake the responsibility of coordinating all treatment efforts, including consultations with specialists."

A communicative doctor can be your lifeline. Good doctors will contact research institutes and universities to find the latest findings and clinical trials that may be happening in your area. Some will even see you are enrolled in such a study, if you are willing.

But no doctor will stand over you, cook or shop for you. As I've said throughout this book - nutrition is the key. There is no substitute for a good, solid diet. The U.S. government recently released diet recommendations tailored to enhance long life and good health: the food pyramid. It is a revision of the old "4 Basic Food Groups" taught for years in health classes.

These dietary guidelines for Americans reflect some of the newest cancer research. The diagram establishes what foods are nutrient-rich and low in fats, and places them at the base of the pyramid: the grains, fruits and vegetables.

How Many Servings Do You Need Each Day?

	Women & some older adults	Children teen girls, active women, most men	Teen boys & active men
Bread group	6	9	11
Vegetable group	3	4	5
Fruit group	2	3	4
Milk group	2-3*	2-3*	2-3*
Meat group	2	2	3

*Women who are pregnant or breastfeeding, teenagers, and young adults to age 24 need 3 servings.

NOTE: The "tip" of The Food Pyramid on the following page shows fat, oils, and sweets. Go easy on these foods because they have a lot of calories from fat and sugars, but few nutrients.

(Source: U.S. Department of Agriculture/U.S. Department of Health and Human Services.)

Food Guide Pyramid
A Guide to Daily Food Choices

Fats, Oil, & Sweets
USE SPARINGLY

KEY - These symbols show that fat and added sugars come mostly from fats, oils and sweets, but can also be part of or added to foods from the other food groups.

■ Fat (naturally occuring and added)

▨ Sugars (added)

Milk, Yogurt, & Cheese Group
2-3 SERVINGS

Meat, Poultry, Fish, Dry Beans, Eggs, & Nuts Group
2-3 SERVINGS

Vegetable Group
3-5 SERVINGS

Fruit Group
2-4 SERVINGS

Bread, Cereal, Rice & Pasta Group
6-11 SERVINGS

HOW TO USE THE DAILY FOOD GUIDE
What Counts As One Serving?

Breads, Cereals, Rice and Pasta
1 slice of bread
1/2 cup of cooked rice or pasta
1/2 cup of cooked cereal
1 ounce of ready-to-eat cereal

Vegetables
1/2 cup of chopped raw or cooked vegetables
1 cup of leafy raw vegetables

Fruits
1 piece of fruit or melon wedge
3/4 cup of juice
1/2 cup of canned fruit
1/4 cup of dried fruit

Milk, Yogurt, and Cheese
1 cup of milk or yogurt
1-1/2 to 2 ounces of cheese

Meat, Poultry, Fish, Dry Beans, Eggs and Nuts
2-1/2 to 3 ounces of cooked lean meat, poultry or fish
Count 1/2 cup of cooked beans, or 1 egg, or 2 tablespoons of peanut butter as 1 ounce of lean meat (about 1/3 serving)

Fats, Oils and Sweets
These are foods such as salad dressings, cream, butter, margarine, sugars, soft drinks, and candies. *Limit calories from these,* especially if you need to lose weight.

NOTE: The amount you eat may be more than one serving. For example, a dinner portion of spaghetti would count as two or three servings of pasta.

(Source: U.S. Department of Agriculture/U.S. Department of Health and Human Services.)

Another helpful change is in food labeling. Nutritional facts are now printed on the labels of most foods, according to FDA regulations enacted in 1993. Consumers can now instantly find the total fat and fiber grams as well as percentages of calcium, sodium, iron and several vitamins.

Shopping for cancer prevention is easier now in the supermarkets. And choosing items rich in nutrition and low in additives sends a message to manufacturers - consumers want foods that are healthy and produced in environmentally friendly ways.

The most striking difference between the "four basic food groups" of the past and the new diagram is protein. The FDA and scientists agree, too much protein is not good. Recommended servings of protein (the "meat group") are scaled back, while grains take a stronger role. (Fats are at the peak of the pyramid, to be eaten only sparingly.)

Many of us were raised by parents who insisted we have meat with every meal. Protein was considered essential for health, but today we know that too much of this important cell-builder can be bad. High protein consumption has been linked to cancer.

WHAT IS PROTEIN?

Mom was right - proteins are very important. We need a good supply to keep our cells healthy and actively reproducing. When we eat proteins, our bodies break them into amino acids - long, complicated strands of molecules that cells use as food. Without them, the body cannot function. Growing bodies - children and adolescents - require more protein than adults.

But protein doesn't have to come from meat. Superior protein sources contain little fat, but supply protein varieties that are more easily broken down and used by body cells.

The Journal of Clinical Nutrition recently produced a chart with revealing percentages of usable energy from various food sources. Red meat wasn't at the top of the chart:

Food Source	Percentage of Usable Energy
fish	62 %
soybeans	45 %
skim milk	40 %
BEEF....................................	38 %
beans and peas	26 %
whole milk	22 %
peanuts	19 %
wheat flour	13 %
rice	8 %
sweet potatoes	4 %

Fish, soybeans and skim milk are the three top protein sources. All three are lower in fat than red meat, too.

When buying dairy products, remember that lowfat milk, yogurt and cheeses are readily available and better for you. Doctors recommend you eat only three eggs per week, and only the egg whites. As much as possible, eliminate cooking oils, butter and margarine. However, be sure to eat the Omega-3 fatty acids contained in linseed oil, safflower oil and soybean oil. Limit garnishes and sauces, and avoid toppings based on egg yolks and mayonnaise.

THE IMPORTANCE OF FIBER

Doctors say you should consume 25 to 30 grams of fiber each day. A high fiber diet is called a "cancer preventive" by the FDA, American Cancer Institute and the American Heart Association. Fiber includes carbohydrates, fruits and vegetables.

Most of our energy comes from carbohydrates. Whole wheat breads, beans, peas and potatoes are good sources of carbohydrates.

Broccoli, cabbage and brussels sprouts are excellent fiber sources because they supply high fiber and help produce cancer-fighting enzymes.

Choose whole and lightly milled grains: rice, barley and buckwheat. Whole-wheat pasta, cereal and crackers are also available.

Beware of processed carbohydrates like white bread, cakes, cookies and boxed macaroni dinners. Unfortunately, the cheapest foods are frequently the most processed. The carbohydrates they supply are stripped of nutritional value through bleaching and other processes. Sauce mixes are usually high in sugar and laced with chemical preservatives.

Fresh fruit is always a good choice - its nutrients haven't been removed through cooking and handling. Unsweetened fruit juices are good, as are unsweetened canned or frozen fruits. If you want cooked fruits or vegetables, simply buy fresh produce and use a steamer with a little water and a short cooking time.

Don't eat jelly, jam or cooked canned or frozen fruit with added sugar. Avoid butter rolls, commercially baked biscuits, muffins, doughnuts, sweet rolls, cakes, egg bread, cheese bread or cake mixes - these usually contain dried eggs and whole milk.

LIPIDS

Lipids are another name for fats - substances the body requires in small amounts. Some lipids are superior to others. They supply a concentrated energy source that delays the emptying of the stomach. They act as insulation for body tissues, and provide a release medium for fat-soluble vitamins. Fats provide structure for brain and nerve tissue. They provide the energy surge we identify with "adrenaline rush" while under stress.

Almost all we hear about fats is bad - mostly because our society overindulges in fat. A little is enough.

OBESITY

One diet-related, and controllable, cancer risk is obesity. This condition is defined as being 10 percent or more above your ideal body weight. It is a risk factor in several diseases - cancer is one of them. An American Cancer Society study of more than 750,000 people found that overweight people face greater risks of cancers of the uterus, stomach and kidneys. An even greater incidence of endometrial, gallbladder, cervical, colic, rectal and breast cancer was reported. The more extra weight you carry, the greater your cancer risk.

Obesity is associated with a 55 percent higher cancer risk in women and a 33 percent increase in risk for men. A 1991 study done at the University of South Florida found that upper-body fat in women increases breast and uterine cancer rates. Women whose fat settles in the stomach area and above usually have more circulating estrogen in their bodies, which may be a factor in some hormone-related cancers.

WHAT CAN YOU DO?

If you are apple-shaped - you tend to carry extra weight in a paunch out front - you should develop a long-term weight reduction plan. Losing even five or ten pounds and keeping it off is better than losing 20 pounds and gaining it all back.

First, be realistic. Set an attainable goal.

Eat less, and in smaller portions. Chew each mouthful of food slowly. Blood sugar levels rise as we eat, and provide that "full" sensation. Those who eat slowly usually eat less.

Eat more complex carbohydrates and fruits and vegetables. Don't eat processed foods.

Exercise regularly. Find a sport that interests you, so you will keep at it.

Chapter XIV

Eminent Doctors & Alternative Cancer Treatments Today

MAX GERSON, MD, AND
NUTRITIONAL METABOLIC THERAPY

Max Gerson was one of the first medical doctors to use nutritional metabolic therapy. Records show many of his patients recovered from cancers and lived out long, healthy lives. His patients included Albert Schweitzer, the Nobel Prize-winning doctor. Schweitzer called Gerson "one of the most eminent medical geniuses in the history of medicine."

"There is no cancer in normal metabolism," Gerson wrote in a case study of 50 patients. Gerson deduced that a combination of degenerated liver and pancreatic functions, bad nutrition and exposure to chemical fertilizers and pollutants causes the body's immune system to break down, giving cancer a foothold. Like other nutritional, metabolic cancer treatments, Gerson focuses on treating the whole person - not just the tumor - through detoxification, nutritional supplements, laetrile and diet.

Dr. Gerson practiced medicine for 52 years, 30 years of those were spent specializing in degenerative disease. The liver was the centerpiece of his therapy - he believed that cancer can be controlled if the liver is healthy. He viewed traditional tumor-specific cancer treatments as treating the symptom, not the root cause.

Like many Eastern practitioners, Gerson believed the healthy body is a balanced system. "A normal body has the capacity to keep all its cells functioning properly," he wrote. "It prevents any abnormal transformation and growth. Therefore, the natural task of a cancer therapy is to bring the body back to that normal physiology, or as near it as possible." Once achieved, it is necessary to keep the metabolism balanced to prevent relapse, he said.

Potassium - or its absence - is a key to bodily balance, Gerson wrote. Potassium is inactive in a sick body, which is quickly overtaken by sodium and related minerals. At the start of his therapy, Gerson concentrated on ridding the body of this sodium buildup while building up its supply of potassium compounds.

Potassium and sodium are "leaders" in two electrically opposite groups of compounds. An imbalance between them results in degeneration of the entire body over many years. Sadly, the patient usually doesn't notice these subtle changes until a major symptom or disease sets in.

Gerson advocated a return to the earth and its processes, including a purification of soil and farmland. "The soil and all that grows in it is not something distant from us," he wrote. "It must be regarded as our external metabolism, which produces the basic substances for our internal metabolism."

Though Dr. Gerson is no longer alive, his therapy lives on through the many doctors who use his therapy and the many patients who continue to recover from cancer. His daughter Charlotte runs the Gerson Institute in Bonita, California, and works closely with patients at the Centro Hospital Internationale del Pacifico in Tijuana, Mexico. This hospital is the international center for Gerson therapy, and draws patients from around the world.

HOW THE THERAPY WORKS

A key to Gerson's therapy is faulty metabolism - the body cannot properly process foods, shuts down its defenses and gets sick. But what causes metabolism to go haywire? Doctors and researchers cite many factors: poor nutrition, pesticide exposure, chemical food additives, cooking methods that destroy food nutrients, depletion of the earth's ozone layer and the increased exposure to ultraviolet light. The list goes on and on.

Metabolic therapies contain two basic components: detoxification and nutritional replacement. Simultaneously, the patient's body must be cleansed of toxins and supplied with nutrients and enzymes that stimulate the immune function, which naturally dissolves tumors.

Nutrients are replaced by a diet rich in whole, natural foods like grains, vegetables and fruits. No foods with additives or preservatives are allowed; coffee, white flour, and sugar are eliminated. Vitamins, minerals and enzymes are added, which strengthen the natural immune system and deactivate toxins produced by tumors.

"Detoxification" describes the process used to flush toxins from the body. These include enemas, gall bladder flushes, and drinking large mugs of herbal teas, and fruit juices.

Another natural method used is enzyme injections. These enzymes are produced in the liver stomach and pancreas, and can break down or activate cancer cells. Cancer patients are usually enzyme-deficient. When their diets are supplemented with enzymes, the protein cell wall that surrounds the tumor is broken down. This allows the white blood cells to attack and kill the cancer. Scientists have known about enzymes' effects on these cell walls for more than a century.

Vaccines and herbal creams are used in some metabolic therapies. The Japanese are developing a substance from native mushrooms that hyper-stimulate the patient's immune system into attacking cancerous growths.

Some doctors report success using oral doses of castor oil, chelation therapy and ozone therapies to detoxify their patients.

In short, metabolic therapy uses many methods to improve overall body functions, instead of focusing on one organ or tumor. The result is a body restored to metabolic balance, and elimination of the conditions that permitted the tumor to develop.

NATURAL CANCER KILLERS

Recent research has found a fascinating new dietary supplement some believe fights cancer. In *The Cancer Chronicles'* Sept. 1993 issue, Dr. Sergejs Kuznetsovs presented a "discovery" known for years in Eastern Europe: the stinkhorn mushroom.

The juice of the mushroom is fermented and taken orally. It has a natural pain-killing effect - and studies find it also reduces the blood marrow-killing effects of the anti-cancer drug 5-FU.

Controversy has swirled around laetrile since the 1950s, when Dr. Ernst Krebs first gave it to patients in his San Francisco clinic. Since then, more than 30 studies have found it safe and effective - but nobody knows how it works.

Many doctors told researchers their patients showed instant, noticeable improvements in their conditions after taking the drug. But the doctors weren't sure if the recovery was due to the laetrile, natural remission or the large doses of vitamins they also took.

The chinese have used laetrile for 2,000 years, and it was known to ancient Greeks, Romans and Persians. Laetrile is a carbohydrate that naturally occurs in chick peas, lentils, lima beans, buckwheat, brown rice, cashews, wheat grass, bean sprouts and apricot and almond seeds. Since the Han Dynasty (206 BC through 220 AD), apricot kernels have been used medically in China to cure coughs, excess phlegm, asthma and constipation.

293

Medicinal use of laetrile is banned in the United States, since the drug did not meet the strict laboratory standards of the Food and Drug Administration.

VITAMINS

Vitamins C, A and E and selenium are given as supplements to stimulate the immune system and cleanse the body of carcinogenic free radicals.

Studies at the National Cancer Society have shown the cancer-fighting properties of vitamin C. Vitamin C increases white blood cell production, and improve cancer patients' survival rates. A study by Nobel prize-winner Dr. Linus Pauling found cancer patients on vitamin C felt better, gained weight and experienced less pain than "regular" patients.

SHARK CARTILAGE

It may seem off-the-wall to look beneath the sea for cancer cures, but some doctors report great success with doses of shark cartilage.

Sharks are exceptionally resistant to water pollution and other marine toxins. The secret of the shark's immunity is in his skeleton: sharks have no bones. Their framework is made of cartilage, which contains no blood vessels. It is made of lipids, proteins, minerals and acids, which act as "angiogenic inhibitors " in other words, they prevent development of blood vessels.

Humans also have cartilage. When humans consume shark cartilage extracts, new blood vessels cannot form. Cancer tumors require new blood vessels to grow and spread - the blood brings the tumor nutrients and carries away its waste products. Stopping vessel development also stops the cancer, and eventually starves it to death. The body's natural disposal system then dissolves and eliminates the tumorous tissue.

Studies at Belgium's Institue Jules Bordet and Rutgers University have proven its effectiveness.

The FDA considers shark cartilage a food supplement, so it is available at many natural food stores.

Some metabolic doctors feel that chemotherapy, radiation and surgery interfere with metabolic healing by destroying some of the body's natural defenses. These orthodox treatments are toxic to the body as a whole. Gerson advised his patients against chemotherapy and radiation, but some metabolic doctors combine traditional therapies with their detoxification and nutritional programs.

HANS NIEPER'S METABOLIC APPROACH

Dr. Hans Nieper, a prominent metabolic doctor from Hanover, Germany, uses this approach. His therapy includes correcting mineral imbalances; use of enzymes to dissolve the mucus layer surrounding tumors; "gene repair therapy," a high-tech method that uses natural substances to change cancer cells' genetic makeup.

Nieper calls his regime "eumatabolic therapy" because he uses natural substances in combination with the body's own metabolism to fight off cancer cells.

DR. NIEPER USUALLY PRESCRIBES:

1. A combination of vitamins, minerals, laetrile, animal and plant extracts, pharmaceutical drugs and vaccines to stimulate the body's natural defense mechanisms. The body's immune system then attacks the cancer. Nieper allows his patients to use orthodox treatments to directly kill the tumor.

2. A vegetarian diet, heavy on whole grain cereals, vegetables and fruits, skim milk and juices, especially carrot juice. He recommends a drastic reduction in consumption of white bread, sugar, cheese and alcohol. Meat, sausage and shellfish are forbidden.

Nieper runs a total blood analysis on all his new patients, and has observed that every one - from children to elders - has mineral deficiencies. He gives patients phosphates, which are full of energy to fight intruding cancer cells. Nieper believes the body stores food energy like a battery, using what it needs throughout the day. It requires special doses of potassium or magnesium to "recharge" itself.

Because zinc is often lacking in cancer patients' blood, Nieper gives his patients zinc and dry beta-carotene supplements. These help white blood cells attack and destroy cancer cells. When these two substances are taken together, the thymus gland is activated. It flashes a signal to the lymphocytes to digest cancer cells. The beta-carotene is taken in dry form, to retain its strong electrical properties. Patients also drink carrot juice mixed with fatty items like cream or butter, which helps this fat-soluble vitamin travel from intestine to blood stream.

FLY TRAPS AND GENE THERAPY

Scientists from throughout the world are working together to map human DNA - or deoxyribonucleic acid - the twisted strands of genetic information contained within every cell. Others alter the cellular information to "program" the cells to change their functions. The technique is now used to alter growth of cancer cells. Dr. Nieper uses this method, too, but uses a natural substance derived from the Venus flytrap plant to change the genetic code.

In 1990, Dr. Helmut Keller developed Carnivora, an extract of this meat-eating jungle plant. It is used to treat AIDS and cancer, and gained notice when former president Ronald Reagan used Carnivora drops following a colon cancer operation.

Nieper uses Carnivora, mistletoe extract and the herb pau d'arco to deactivate the genetic information sent out by Oncogenes - an unstable gene group found in the cells of patients with cancer. Some scientists think Oncogenes descend from viruses that enter the body as an infection, or they are inherited from a parent. They are present in every body, but usually remain inactive.

296

NIEPER'S DIET

Preferred foods: oatmeal, millet, whole grain bread
skim milk
fish, in limited quantities
fruit and fibrous vegetables
carrot juice
enzyme preparations
"omniflora" capsules

Restricted foods: meat and sausages
cheese
sugar
pastries and puddings
shell fish
alcohol
"junk beverages" like soda and Kool-Aid
apple juice (it's high in glucose)
distilled water

Nieper's patients aren't to drink alcohol or eat meat or dairy products, because all increase mucus production. He believes it is the same mucus that coats and protects cancer tumors. In addition, animals are given synthetic hormones in their feed to hasten their trip to market or increase milk production. Nieper believes these hormones contaminate the products made from the cattle who eat them.

Nieper also believes average doctors and oncologists aren't aware of the latest cancer treatments, and frequently patients aren't given the treatment they need in time. He cites a wide gap between new cancer research and the practice of everyday medicine, and blames it on bureaucracies and government agencies that take years to approve new drugs and therapies.

RESEARCH SUPPORTS NIEPER'S TREATMENTS

Dr. Nieper incorporates the latest research into his therapy. DHEA, a natural blood steroid, is prescribed to Nieper's cancer patients as an aid to detoxification. Studies show that DHEA in the blood causes some cancers to go into remission.

Nieper also prescribes shark liver oil. This slippery substance contains squalene, a substance that removes sodium from the body and gives sharks a remarkable immunity to cancer and carcinogens. Scientists at the Smithsonian Institution in Washington, D.C., studied 25,000 sharks that inhabit polluted waters. They found only one malignant tumor in the lot.

People with cancer almost always have high levels of sodium in their tissues. When dosed with shark liver oil, this excess is purged from the body.

Thymus injections are also administered. These activate enzymes that dissolve cancer cells. The shots also contain zinc and dry beta-carotene, which stimulate cancer-fighting white blood cells.

Although some other metabolic therapies frown on traditional surgical, radiation and chemotherapies, Nieper sees them as valuable tools - adjuncts to a whole-body approach.

"Chemotherapy might have a beneficial effect in co-operation with the much more important immunological and eumetabolic methods of treating cancer," Nieper wrote in his book "Revolution." "One thing is certain - chemotherapy can produce positive results of lasting value only when it is encouraged by a strong 'tailwind' from the body's own immune defense system. Chemotherapy must never be so extensive that valuable mechanisms of the body's own defenses are thoughtlessly damaged."

KATHERINE MAYER'S MIRACULOUS CANCER RECOVERY

In 1985, 65-year-old Katherine Mayer was told by her

California doctor that she had incurable bone cancer. She was given two years to live.

A few months later, after her weight dropped to 79 pounds, Katherine heard of Dr. Nieper at a convention of the Cancer Control Society. She and her husband immediately headed to Germany to find him.

Katherine was admitted to Silbersee Hospital in Hanover, and immediately began the Nieper therapy. She took calcium for her bones, calcium 2-AEP to protect her cell membranes from her immune system, and shark liver oil and vitamin C to cut off blood supplies to the cancerous cells.

After two weeks of therapy, diets and injections of thymus extract, magnesium supplements and laetrile, Katherine went home. She already felt better, she said. She could walk more freely, and the pain had decreased.

Six months later, Katherine returned to Germany. Nieper adjusted her medications and tailored her diet to her healing body.

In August 1990, five years after he gave Katherine two years to live, her family doctor ran diagnostic tests on his "miracle patient." Katherine Mayer was cancer-free.

Katherine still is on the semi-vegetarian diet Nieper prescribed. She takes thymus shots and several vitamin pills each day. She expects to live into her 80s, she said, and when her time comes, she doesn't plan to die of cancer.

THE ISSELS WHOLE-BODY THERAPY

Dr. Josef Issels also uses a combination of therapies to successfully drive cancer into remission while building up the body's natural immunity. His therapy includes anti-tumor vaccines, a low-protein diet, "fever therapy," and the now-familiar cleansing and rebuilding process.

If you read about the Livingston Therapy in chapter 4, the Issel method will seem familiar: he believes that a deteriorated immune system gives a foothold to a "live oncogenic agent" - a microbe that feeds on wastes given off by cancer tumors. Similar to Livingston's cancer bacteria theory, this microbe can change form and go into the body tissues, laying in wait for opportunities to return to its original state.

Issels claims the body has four interrelated defense systems. If any one malfunctions, a tumor may result. These systems are:

- The lymphocytes and antibodies
- The detoxifying organs: large intestines, kidneys, liver and skin
- The epithelial tissue, which lines body cavities with "friendly" bacteria
- The connective tissues, which store protein, salts and water and bind and destroy toxins and microbes

Issels' treatments work to purify and restore all four systems to cooperative functioning. He uses:

- Detoxification
- Ozone therapy
- Homeopathic remedies
- Liver extract injections
- Enzyme supplements
- Psychotherapy
- Low-dose chemotherapy or radiation - when patient's life is endangered

Studies performed in England and Holland of Issel's patients found that 16 to 17 percent of those previously diagnosed as terminally ill now lead normal, cancer-free lives. Dr. John Anderson, author of the London study, wrote, "I am of the considered opinion that this is a new approach to cancer treatment and appears to be a considerable improvement over what is usually offered. My overall opinion is that Issels approach to cancer treatment is a unique and pioneering solution to a difficult problem. He is undoubtingly producing clinical remissions in patients who have been regarded as hopeless."

FEVER THERAPY, OR "HYPOTHERMIA"

Dr. Issels uses carefully monitored hyperthermia with his cancer patients. "Sweat therapy" has been used for hundreds of years in Europe. It causes a dramatic increase in white blood counts, which in turn fight off disease and produce bacteria-killing antibodies. Issels administers monthly "fever shots" to patients, inducing a high fever for up to five hours. Heat kills cancer cells. In 1984, the federal Food and Drug Administration gave its stamp of approval to the practice as a medical cancer treatment.

The National Cancer Institute stated in its "Cancer Weekly" in 1989 that heat therapy increases the effectiveness of other treatments by 25 to 35 percent. Very good results have been seen in cancers of the brain, breast, neck and skin.

OZONE THERAPY

Issels also uses ozone therapy to increase the amount of oxygen in patients' bloodstreams. Cancer cannot live or reproduce in an oxygen-rich environment, but healthy cells thrive there.

Ozone therapy works thus: Issels draws a volume of blood from the patient, combines it with an ozone-oxygen mixture, and puts the enriched blood back into the patient's body. This creates a distinctly unfriendly environment for cancer.

Issels also employs "substitution therapy" in his cancer treatment, an age-old homeopathic technique that supposedly restores health to specific organs. He gives his patients organ extracts - liver extract for liver patients, for instance, to build up immunity and restore balance.

ISSELS' DIET

Diet is critical in changing body chemistry. As you might expect by now, this diet is heavy on fresh fruit and vegetables - they comprise about 3/4 of this diet. Issels believes cancer patients need lots of fluids, so he has them drink large amounts of water, juices and herbal teas.

Issels dispenses few vitamin and mineral supplements, but he swears by vitamins A, B complex, C and E. Some proteins, like buttermilk and cottage cheese, are permitted on his diet, but meats are prohibited as too hard to digest. Yogurt and supplements of lactobacillus acidophilus are recommended, too - they encourage the growth of "friendly" intestinal bacteria.

RIGHT DOWN TO THE TEETH

Bad teeth and tonsils are removed under Issels' program, too, in an effort to "eliminate all causal factors." The doctor caused a splash in 1987 in New York, when he told practitioners that cancer patients should have all amalgam fillings removed from their teeth. A controversy erupted in the medical community, but Dr. F. Fuller Royal, medical director of the Nevada Clinic, said that metal fillings have been known to be toxic since the late 1800s.

"It's not out of the realm of possibility that dental metals are related to an increase in cancer in the U.S. today," Royal said. "Continuous exposure to small electric currents, as occurs with amalgams, is known to stress the endocrine glands, decrease immune system activity and may enhance certain viruses and bacteria."

Movies and videos of Issels' patients don't show hospital beds, monitors and feeding tubes - they feature lines of hearty folk carefully scaling mountain trails at his Alpine Ringburg Clinic. Issels insisted his patients get outdoors and take in fresh air and exercise.

WHERE PATIENTS CAN FIND ISSELS PRACTITIONERS

Dr. Ahmed Elkadi studied under Issel, and opened his cancer clinic on the Gulf Coast of Florida in 1984. About half his patients show improvements, he says, and some have remissions. Most stay at the clinic for intensive treatments for up to three months, then go home to follow a special diet. The clinic can be contacted at:

Panama City Clinic
Ahmed Elkadi, MD
236 South Tyndall Parkway
Panama City, FL 32404
Phone 904-763-7689

Dr. Wolfgang Woeppel, a German MD, is one of Issels prize pupils. He can be contacted at:

Hufeland Klinik
Wolfgang Woeppel, MD
Bismarckstrasse
Bad Mergentheim, Germany
Phone 011-49-7931-8185

WILLIAM KELLY'S NUTRITIONAL-METABOLIC THERAPY

Dr. William D. Kelly is a dentist in Texas. In 1965, after his doctor diagnosed him with terminal pancreatic cancer, Kelly used a longtime interest in nutrition to design his own impromptu therapy - and sent his cancer into remission. His recovery led him to further investigate the role of proper diet and nutrition in cancer treatment, and eventually led to his developing a "nutritional-metabolic" therapy.

Kelly's patients undergo detoxification, special diets and supplements of pancreatic enzymes. Although his treatment hadn't received widespread acceptance among orthodox doctors, it has gained credibility in the hands of Dr. Nicholas Gonzalez, a New York City physician.

Gonzalez' 500-page study of Kelly's patients was hailed as "the finest case review ever conducted concerning alternative cancer therapy." Dr. Harold Ladas, a Hunter College biologist, said "Gonzalez has given us convincing evidence that diet and nutrition produce long-term remission in cancer patients, almost all of whom were beyond conventional help."

Kelly's popularity peaked in 1969, with the publication of "One Answer to Cancer," a layman's outline of his theories. Its bestseller status created alarm among the Texas Medical Society. The doctors' group launched an investigation into Kelly's methods. Undercover agents pretended to be cancer patients to see up close how the therapy worked. Although no unauthentic medical data or false records were found, the medical society obtained a restraining order that forbade Kelly to treat any "non-dental disease." His publisher was ordered to withdraw Kelly's book from the market. In 1971, Kelly's therapy appeared on the American Cancer Society's list of "unproven treatments."

Nevertheless, patients continued to search him out. In 1980, actor Steve McQueen was suffering from inoperable lung cancer. He entered a Mexican hospital where Kelly's therapy was practiced. He claimed to follow the strict diets, but continued smoking cigarettes and eating junk food. Still, his tumor stopped growing. After eight weeks on the Kelly therapy he was able to stop taking pain killers and had gained several pounds.

An enthusiastic McQueen signed himself out of the hospital a week later, and immediately returned to his old lifestyle and diet. He died a year later.

KELLY'S VIEW OF CANCER

Dr. Kelly believed the cause of cancer is a bodily inability to break down and use protein. Tumors occur because of this metabolic problem, he said. Even if the tumor is removed, the cancer will likely return if the underlying metabolism problem is not treated.

The pancreas is the key to breaking down proteins, he taught. Those deficient in pancreatic enzymes are good targets for cancer, since these chemicals are the body's first line of defense against cancer cells.

Cancer creates mineral imbalances, Kelly said, which contribute to tumor growth by impairing the immune system. Kelly believed that some bodies oxidize food more quickly than others, and require more meat proteins to operate. Each patient's regime is tailored to his own unique metabolism.

Raw, organically grown vegetables - easily digested - figure big in his diet, while complex proteins are virtually eliminated. Supplements, up to 150 per day, are prescribed. They include vitamins and minerals, enzymes and concentrates of raw beef organs and glands. Kelly thought these contain tissue-growth factors and hormones that are natural cancer defenses.

His theories are upheld by research. When patients are given enzymes, the chemicals seem to head straight for cancerous tumors and "digest" the affected tissue. This breakdown releases large amounts of cancer cell debris through the bloodstream, which creates a temporary toxic effect until the liver and kidneys can filter out the debris. This is why Kelly suggests patients give their bodies a rest after a large enzyme dose, to let their body's "filters" catch up with the detoxification process.

Other "detox" methods include daily coffee enemas, which stimulate the liver and gallbladder to release large amounts of waste into the bowel. Most of the waste eliminated is enzyme inhibitors. Frequent enemas prevent suppression of protein-digesting enzymes, which eat away at the tumors' mucous coat and make them vulnerable to the body's immune mechanisms.

Kelly also employed techniques familiar to those in "12-step" recovery programs. He helped patients accept their disease while giving them hope for recovery. He urged belief in a force greater than self - a "higher power." His patients were helped to let go of negative thought patterns and behaviors and establish positive habits of soul-searching and acceptance.

The Kelly treatment has some powerful supporters. Pat Judson, one of Kelly's success stories, now heads the Metro Detroit chapter of the Foundation for Advancement of Cancer Therapy, or FACT. Judson told a committee of the Michigan State Legislature, "If I had accepted the advice of my doctor, if I had not been directed to Dr. Kelly, I would be another cancer statistic."

Kelly doesn't promise miracles, but he claims a 50 percent success rate for patients whose doctors have given them three months to live. For those with more advanced cancers, the rate drops to 25 percent. But as FACT director Ruth Sackman told the state lawmakers, "enough of Kelly's patients who lived ten years or more suggest a pattern of survival. They indicate that he uses a sound system."

A closer look at the Gonzalez study reveals a median survival rate of pancreatic cancer - one of the deadliest varieties - was nine years. Some of these patients are still living today. Statistics like these are unheard of in conventional cancer therapy.

The Mutual Benefit Life Insurance Company recently evaluated the Gonzalez report, visited former patients and several clinics and drew up a written report of their own. Robert Maver, vice president and researcher, wrote "The results are indeed extraordinary. This is a prime example of an innovative therapy that merits evaluation, but is being ignored. As costly as cancer is to our industry, and in light of such promising, cost-effective preliminary results, our industry should consider funding such a trial."

Those interested in detailed information on the Kelly Therapy should contact:

Nicholas Gonzalez, M.D.
737 Park Ave.
New York, NY 10021
Phone 212-213-3337

CORNELIUS MOERMAN'S ANTI-CANCER DIET

Dr. Cornelius Moerman was pioneer in the dietary approach to cancer treatment. During the 1930's, when most doctors still believed in the "cellular hypothesis" of cancer, Moerman was the first to declare the disease stemmed from an overall breakdown of the immune system. He identifies three "irritants" that are responsible for cancer: pollution, radiation and improper nutrition. Each of these, the doctor said, can effect cellular DNA and create cancer.

Moerman identified the most effective anti-cancer nutrients as vitamins A, C and E. He believed that a body in decay created an oxygen shortage on the cellular level. These starved cells would adapt to their conditions, and begin to use glucose - sugar - to produce energy. It is this process that produces sugar cravings during times when the body really craves vitamin-rich foods. The body knows it can use fermentation to turn a candy bar into a sudden energy burst. But the food is devoid of real nutritional value, and the immune system isn't built up.

In addition, recent research proves that cancer seems to thrive in a sugar-rich, oxygen-poor environment.

Healthy cells get energy and oxygen through a variety of nutrients found in organically grown foods. Moerman believed that tumors are visible signs that the body has adapted itself to producing energy by fermenting sugars rather than oxidizing nutritional foods. Tumors occur in the organs most vulnerable to an immune system breakdown, he theorized, and the body's general weakness gave the cancer a free rein to spread and grow.

MOERMAN'S VIEW OF CANCER

Cancer is not an autonomous, local disease with power to destroy the body.

Faulty nutrition which influences metabolism precedes formation of cancer tissue.

Cancer cannot gain a foothold in a healthy body.

Moerman owed the genesis of his cancer theories to a neighbor boy's pet pigeon. The bird had developed a tumor. Moerman extracted some cancer tumors from the pigeon and injected them into a healthy pigeon. The sick pigeon died (Moerman bought the boy a new one), but the other pigeon remained healthy. From this the doctor concluded that cancer cannot be introduced into a healthy body.

He studied pigeons and nutrition for ten years, testing for nutritional elements that seemed to promote optimal health. Through this research he found his "eight vital substances:" vitamins A, C, E, B-complex, citric acid, iodine, iron and sulphur.

Moerman got to try his new theory on a human subject in 1939, when Lenndert Brinkman came to him with terminal stomach cancer. Brinkman volunteered to try Moerman's new treatment, figuring he had little to lose. After a year of "eight vital substance" supplements and "truckloads of oranges and lemons," Brinkman's cancer was gone. He lived into his 90s.

Moerman refined his methods and dosages as years passed, and eventually identified 17 common cancer symptoms:

MOERMAN'S CANCER WARNING SIGNS

1. Dry skin, with considerably reduced elasticity; associated symptoms include excessively calloused feet and discolored facial skin
2. Aberrations with mucous membranes
3. Chapped and sore mouth corners
4. Red spots and scaly skin on and around the nose
5. Dull, brittle nails and chapped hands
6. Brown, furry coating on tongue
7. Thin, lifeless hair
8. Gums that bleed easily
9. Black bruises that result from minor bumps

10. Wounds that heal slowly, if at all
11. Formation of jelly-like regeneration tissue in a wound or healing surgical incision.
12. Fatigue without due reason
13. Pale complexion
14. Cravings for sour foods
15. Apathy, listlessness and a loss of interest in hobbies and pursuits that once were fascinating
16. Low energy
17. Sudden weight loss

MOERMAN'S DIET AND SUPPLEMENTS

FOODS PERMITTED:

GRAINS: whole grain bread, pasta, crackers; unpolished brown rice, barley, oat bran, wheat germ; wheat, oat and corn flakes.

DAIRY: butter, buttermilk, cream cheese, cottage cheese, egg yolk, lowfat milk, sour cream, yogurt.

VEGETABLES: all vegetables are permitted, and should be eaten raw or lightly steamed. Exceptions are: beans, red or white potatoes, sweet potatoes, cabbage and sauerkraut.

FRUIT: All fresh fruits are allowed except the following: dates, figs, sweet grapes and rhubarb. (Fruit juices are highly recommended, especially carrot, beet and orange juice mixed with lemon.)

FORBIDDEN FOODS:

White flour and anything that contains white flour: bread, pasta, pudding, cakes, biscuits, gravy, cookies and sauces.

Cheese with high fat and salt content: blue, brie, cheddar, Munster, Swiss.

Egg white, coffee, cocoa, alcohol, fish, meat, shellfish, margarine, mushrooms, vegetable shortening and hydrogenated vegetable oils, beans, peas, lentils, kidney beans, animal fats, chemical preservatives, broths made of fish, meat or shellfish, caffeinated teas, refined white sugar and its products.

Cigars, cigarettes and other types of tobacco are also verboten.

SAMPLE DAILY MENU

Breakfast:	Juice of two oranges and a lemon Whole grain bread with butter or cheese, OR Oatmeal with fruit and lowfat milk Buttermilk Herb tea
Mid-morning:	Apple juice mixed with beet juice Fruit
Lunch:	Brown rice or whole grain pasta Steamed vegetables Butter pat Mixed salad with lemon juice dressing Fruit
Mid-afternoon:	One or two egg yolks blended with 1 cup lowfat milk Buttermilk with grape juice Whole-grain crackers
Dinner:	Whole pea soup Whole-grain bread Raw vegetables Yogurt Fruit Buttermilk
Late evening:	Buttermilk with juice of 1 lemon
Bedtime:	Warm lowfat milk

310

RESEARCH SUPPORTS MOERMAN'S THEORY

In 1954, Dr. Wim Romijn wrote an essay called "Health and Prosperity" that outlined a startling discovery: the Nazi occupation of Holland during World War II seemed to send cancer statistics plummeting. After the war ended, cancer rates went back up again.

Romijn felt the dip in cancer was a direct result of the anti-cancer effects of Hitler's compulsory diet.

Those who lived through the occupation survived on corn bread and rye bread - white bread disappeared from the market. Sugar, tea and coffee were not available. There was no margarine, and alcohol production slowed to a trickle. Meat and dairy products were rare treats.

Romijn felt that "prosperity" and the diet of the prosperous could lead to poor health and eventual cancer. His findings supported Moerman, whose diet is similar to that wartime fare.

Years later, British and Dutch biochemists discovered and named "anticarcinogens," substances that can attack cancer cells. These substances halt the enzyme-like activity of carcinogens on cell DNA, which in turn stops the rapid growth of cancer cells.

Vitamin A - one of Moerman's "vital substances" is an important anti-carcinogen. The Dutch scientists found it could turn malignant cancers to benign in laboratory tests. After an extensive 1983 pharmaceutical study, Moerman's therapy was named a bona fide cancer treatment by the Dutch Ministry of Health.

Other researchers, including Linus Pauling, MD, testify to other aspects of Moerman's theory. Pauling's research on the effects of Vitamin C on tumors mentions Moerman and his pioneering theory.

TRADITIONAL CANCER TREATMENTS
BASED ON OUTDATED THEORY

Most 20th century cancer treatments are outdated. They are based on the theories of a 19th century Prussian pathologist Rudolph Virchow, whose 1858 theory was considered a breakthrough in its time. His five-point process followed a pattern:

1. Cancer is a localized disease
2. Cancer manifests itself in tumor form
3. Tumors are made of abnormal cells
4. Cancer cell multiplication is autonomous and un- stoppable
5. The cells distinguish themselves by their infiltrating growth

Virchow's theories don't hold up to current research on immune-deficient diseases and environmental toxins. We know that many factors, like diet and nutritional supplements, effect cancerous tumors, and that the disease can be prevented by following dietary guidelines.

The National Cancer Institute and the Federal Food and Drug Administration agree that diet effects cancer, and have developed lifestyle and dietary recommendations for Americans concerned about cancer.

But even with such heavy evidence against it, Virchow's theory is still followed in standard cancer treatment. Orthodox oncologists still focus on the tumor only, following the belief that cancer is a localized disease. Even after using radiation, chemical poisons and surgeries, tumors frequently return, or turn up elsewhere in the body. The patient's body is poisoned and worn down by these treatments, less able to fight off infections or new cancers.

Even worse, the patient is taught to look outside himself for answers and cures, when the answers are inside. While cancer patients who opt for traditional treatments spend their energy (and money) looking to technology for a cure, they could use the same resources to examine their diet and lifestyles and make needed changes without so much pain, indignity and expense.

METABOLIC NUTRITIONAL THERAPIES: THE WHOLE APPROACH

Metabolic Therapies, as a whole, stress treating the entire person, not just the cancer. The doctor looks at the patient's diet and lifestyle to find what is causing their immune system to malfunction. The patient is deeply involved in his own treatment. He is listened-to and heard. Together the patient and doctor work together to find what changes must be made.

After a special diet and supplement schedule is agreed on, the patient learns to listen to his own body, to accept the disease as a symptom, not a dead end. Patients feel in control and involved, and are encouraged to seek the support of others who face similar situations.

Most cancer patients who look to these therapies live longer than those on traditional therapies. All of them live their last years drug-free, with much less pain and a sense of participation in their own treatment.

BIOLOGICAL AND PHARMACOLOGIC THERAPIES

ANTINEOPLASTIN THERAPY

Dr. Stanislaw Burzynski, a Polish biochemist, discovered this anti-cancer treatment while researching the short chains of amino acids the body produces - called "peptides." These acids are part of the body's biochemical defense mechanism, a blood-based defense that is separate from the immune system. These chemicals don't attack or destroy defective cells, they reprogram and correct them by changing the cells' genetic codes - similar to the way cancer operates.

"The body itself has this treatment for cancer," Burzynski said. He found that cancer patients are short of peptides - possessing only 2 to 3 percent the normal, healthy amount. When he introduced these compounds into the blood-streams of cancer patients, their tumors shrank. Some even had complete remissions.

Thousands of cancer patients have found relief since Burzynski opened his clinic in 1977. The therapy works on almost all types of cancer, and seems even to work better on cancer types that are resistant to radiation, chemotherapy and immunotherapy: cancers of the brain, prostate, lung, bladder and pancreas.

In 1991, Burzynski told his colleagues at the International Congress of Chemotherapy about results of trials with 20 patients who had astrocytoma, a virulent form of brain tumor. He treated all with antineoplastins after all other forms of cancer therapies had failed.

Four patients experienced complete remission.

Ten showed stabilization, with most tumors reducing in size by 50 percent or more.

About 1 year after the study, several of these ten had complete or partial remissions.

THE THEORY

Burzynski isolated 119 "messenger peptides" that bond to cancer cells and feed them chemical information needed to convert back to normal cell functioning. He was convinced that "cancer is a disease of information processing." All peptides are messengers, and all of them accomplish their mission: telling cells what to do. By sending doses of these peptides into the blood stream, the renegade cells infected with cancer may be influenced to normal functioning again.

IN PRACTICE

Ryan Werthwein was 10 years old when doctors found he had inoperable thalamic glioblastoma, a brain tumor.

He was given six to nine months to live, but underwent five weeks of radiation therapy nevertheless. The radiation had no effect on the cancer, but it devastated the boy's mental functioning and stunted his growth. Disgusted by their treatment by the medical establishment, Ryan's parents looked into alternative treatments.

In April 1990, Ryan started antineoplastin therapy. A month later, the tumor mass broke down, and his condition began to steadily improve. The Werthweins were elated. "It felt as if a miracle had occurred," Sharon Werthwein said.

An MRI scan done four weeks after his treatment began showed barely-visible tumor remnants. By November 1, Ryan was in complete remission.

Sharon Werthwein is understandably enthusiastic. "The thing that attracted us to Dr. Burzynski's approach is that it's safe and nontoxic, without the horrendous damage and pain that chemotherapy and radiation cause. Besides, we figured "Our boy is dying. What have we got to lose by trying this method."

Ryan still receives antineoplastin treatment through a small infusion pump worn on his belt. He is fully mobile, and has no pain or discomfort.

THE THERAPY

Antineoplastin is administered orally or through a catheter, during outpatient visits to Burzynski's clinic that go on from three months to a year. The therapy is expensive, with most of the cost going to the drugs that are specially manufactured at the clinic. (No major pharmaceutical company has agreed to try making the substances.) Fortunately, many medical insurance plans cover the cost at least partially.

GASTON NAESSENS AND 714-X THERAPY

Gaston Naessens is a French-Canadian biologist who discovered a somewhat backward-appearing cancer treatment that actually feeds cancer cells with nitrogen-enriched camphor compound called 714-X.

Naessens spent 40 years as a bio-researcher before discovering the "somatid," a microbe he believes is an early ancestor of DNA. Every living thing is aswim in somatids, which determine the genetic makeup of the organism they live in. Naessens studied hundreds of somatid cultures in his laboratory, and found the microbes take on 16 different cycles of life as a disease like cancer progresses within the body and the immune system is weakened and overcome.

The biologist realized this could be an important diagnostic tool. Doctors could tell how far a disease had progressed by observing which form a patient's somatids had taken. Cancer tumors form, Naessens says, when somatids revert to primitive forms, feed on sugars and begin to multiply rapidly - usually when the immune system is somehow weakened. These tumors crave nitrogen, which it takes from supply the body usually carries to maintain healthy tissue. The rest of the body then is robbed of many nutrients.

Tumors produce a substance Naessens calls CKF, or "K Factor," which paralyzes the body's immune system. The cancer grows unchecked. Stopping this process became Naessen's mission.

NAESSEN'S THERAPY

After years of experimenting, Naessens found a compound that shuts down the tumor's production of CKF, in turn allowing the immune system to return to work. He called his compound 714-X.

714-X is nontoxic. It provides nitrogen to the cancer cells, so the patient's own nutritional supply is not compromised. Because the cancer is getting the nitrogen it needs, the process used to create CKF is shut down. The rejuvenated immune system then recognizes the cancer as an intruder and kills it.

316

Naessens is not a medical doctor, but he has advised many doctors on the use of 714-X for cancer treatment. The usual prescription is three 21-day periods of daily injections, with three-day resting periods between each of the cycles. Treatment is prolonged for patients with advanced cancer.

Dr. Warren Harrison, a Washington, D.C. medical doctor, uses 714-X in his practice. He reports that six cancer patients treated with the compound reported increased strength, appetite, energy and calm, followed by tumor shrinkage and pain relief.

Those interested in more information on Naessen's therapy can contact:

Centre d' Orthobiologie
Somatidienne de l'Estrie (COSE)
5270 Fontaine
Rock Forest, Quebec J1N 3B6
Canada
Phone 819-564-7883

Genesis Clinic
West Provida
PO Box 3460
Chula Vista, CA 91902-0004
Phone 619-424-9552
(clinic located in Tijuana, Mexico)

REVICI THERAPY

Dr. Emanuel Revici treats cancer with lipids, an organic, non-toxic form of chemotherapy.

Revici was born in Romania, and practices medicine in New York City. His theories have for more than 60 years been applied to diseases like cancer, schizophrenia, allergies, burns, addiction, AIDS and Alzheimer's.

Revici sees health as a balance between opposing forces: Anabolic, or building-up; and Catabolic, or breaking down.

Revici says that predominance of one over the other leads to disease.

THE THEORY BEHIND THE THERAPY

Revici believes the body's defense system passes through four chemical stages when fighting a major disease. One stage cannot begin until the previous stage is finished. If any one of the stages breaks down, lipids or sterols build up and overturn the body's anabolic or catabolic levels, and the defense system cannot move on to the next level. The doctor says most chronic diseases are characterized by these abnormal processes. Over time, the imbalance can lead to cancer.

TREATMENT

Revici uses urinalysis to analyze patient's lipid levels and determine the number of fatty acids and sterols in the blood, and then administers tailored lipid-based compounds to normalize the imbalance. He calls this "biologically-guided chemotherapy."

The doctor says cancer tumors are very rich in free lipids, and readily take up the compounds he administers. Some are synthetic compounds that bear trace elements - like selenium - that are toxic to tumor tissue. This therapy was successfully used through 1983 at St. Louis Veteran's Administration Hospital.

Other success stories include Marianne Dimetres, who faced complicated surgery in 1988 after doctors found she had Stage 4 uterine cancer. Dimetres refused the operation, and began Dr. Revici's guided lipid therapy and a wheatgrass diet. (Found elsewhere in this book.) Tests conducted in 1991 found no cancer in her system.

"I strongly believe you should have total control of our own healing and the freedom to choose what's best for you," Dimetres said.

318

HYDRAZINE SULFATE: FROM ROCKET FUEL TO CANCER CURE

The industrial chemical hydrazine sulfate has been a friend to industry for many years - rocketeers used it for fuel during World War II. In the early 1970's, a researcher named Joseph Gold proposed it be used as a cancer therapy. Since then, reams of research have piled up in support of this chemical's anti-cancer effects.

Cancer thrives in a sugar-rich environment. Gold put this theory to work on lab rats, and tried hydrazine sulfate injections to see what effect it would have on the cancerous rodents.

Gold found the chemical stopped the flow of new glucose (blood sugar) from the liver. The tumor eventually "starved" for lack of new glucose, while the body stopped the wasting away so typical of late cancer.

In 1975, Gold showed that hydrazine sulfate also enhances the effects of conventional anti-cancer drugs. He claimed that a combination of chemotherapy and hydrazine sulfate could treat cancer.

Later that year, Gold tried his ideas on 84 terminally ill cancer patients. The results showed that 70 percent of the patients said they felt better, had increased appetite, weight gain and less pain. 17 percent showed physical signs of improvement, like measurable tumor regression or disappearance of cancer symptoms.

A 1987 UCLA study found that hydrazine sulfate can improve the body's efficiency in calorie distribution in the final stage of cancer, and can curb the tendency to "waste away" as the disease progresses. After a month of hydrazine therapy, 83 percent of the sampled patients had gained weight and kept it on. Their appetites improved, and their bodies better digested and utilized the food they ate.

A team of 11 researchers at the Petrov Research Institute of Oncology in St. Petersburg worked on hydrazine sulfate therapy since the 1970s. More than 740 patients with five

319

different types of cancer were treated and evaluated. Half the patients had less weight loss, muscle weakness and wasting symptoms. Fourteen percent had "extremely good" results; 33 percent had "moderately good" benefits. Ten percent had tumor regressions.

Three major studies identified the cancers that are most responsive to the chemical: desmosarcoma, neuroblastoma, laryngeal and breast cancers, and Hodgkin's Disease.

The National Cancer Institute is now conducting a Phase 3 clinical trial of hydrazine sulfate on cancer at three medical centers.

ESSAIC: A CANCER TREATMENT FROM THE CANADIAN WOODS

Essiac is an herbal mixture made famous by Renee Caisse, a Canadian nurse, during the 1920s and '30s. Caisse obtained the medicine in 1922 from a patient who said the formula cured her of breast cancer. It was given to her by an Ojibway medicine man.

Although hundreds of cancer cures were documented, the Canadian medical establishment forced Caisse out of business in the early 1940's. Her formula was never accepted by most doctors, but hopeless patients continued to stream to Caisse's little house in Ontario.

In 1959, Caisse traveled to Boston to work at the prestigious Brusch Medical Center. There her formula gained credence as doctors found it decreased tumor masses, changes in cell formations and brought a cessation of pain to dozens of patients.

The nurse's formula is a simple one: It contains sheep sorrel, burdock root, rhubarb root and slippery elm bark in a water base and as a tea. It is now available in health food stores in the United States and Canada under the name Flor-Essence.

CANCELL

CanCell is a non-toxic cancer treatment developed by Jim Sheridan, an attorney and chemist from Pittsburgh.

Sheridan says he doesn't know all the active substances in his anti-cancer formula, but that it contains a natural catechol - a chemical that stops respiration. His theory involves cutting off the flow of energy to cancer cells and forcing them to take a "primitive form," which is then killed by the immune system.

Sheridan says he's fought an uphill battle with the American Cancer Society, the FDA and the Biosciences division of Battelle Institute in Columbus to get his formula medical testing and recognition. For many years he gave the medicine away to those who asked for it.

Even now, Sheridan warns patients the medicine is not a cure for cancer, only a way to instruct the body to fight cancer as if it were a foreign invader.

CanCell continues to be a great unknown in alternative cancer treatment. But many patients continue to seek out Sheridan and his CanCell medicine.

To receive CanCell, contact:

Ed Sopcak
P.O. Box 496
Howell, Michigan 48843
Phone 313-684-5529
Monday through Friday, between 11:00 a.m. and
2:00 p.m. Eastern Standard Time

ENDERLEIN THERAPY

Dr. Guenther Enderlein, a bacteriologist, has developed a biological cancer therapy based on 60 years of study of live blood plasma.

When a patient comes to him, Enderlein takes a sample of his blood and carefully watches it through a microscope.

321

By watching how it changes over time, he can supposedly tell the state of the patient's health and draw up a treatment plan.

Enderlein's theory is based on the acid/alkaline balance of normal blood. Cancer patients usually have high alkaline levels. When the balance is restored, cancer cells revert to a microorganism form, Enderlein says.

The doctor uses diet, detoxification methods and lifestyle changes to change the body's PH level. Because cancer lives on nitrogen, potassium, calcium and iron, patients are given a diet low in these nutrients. They are encouraged to increase their oxygen intake through exercise and diet. They're advised to stop smoking and avoid exposure to pollutants.

Chapter XV
Forewarned Is Forearmed

"That man is wise who gains his wisdom from the experience of another."

Titus Maccius Plautus, a Roman philosopher and playwright who lived from 254 to 184 B.C., penned those words over two thousand years ago. They are as fresh and true today as they were when the Roman empire ruled the world. Given the fact that killing disease rampages through our modern and civilized society today, perhaps they are even more pertinent to our time than to that of Plautus.

This book is rich in the experiences of others. We have presented the research of medical scientists world-wide and detailed some remarkable stories of ordinary people who have followed healthful regimens which many times brought them back from the edge of the grave itself. Science *is* making progress, but very slowly, against cancer. But what we must not do is wait complacently for a cure. We cannot afford to rest securely in the arms of medical science thinking that a cure will be found in time to save us. The following facts will show you very graphically exactly why:

PREVENTION IS VITAL

TESTING THE STATISTICS — Three prestigious medical research institutions (The Sloan-Kettering Cancer Center, The Mayo Clinic, and Johns Hopkins University) collaborated in a study of over 30,000 middle-aged men who were heavy smokers and therefore considered at risk of developing lung cancer. This research involved intensive and regular screening of half the men, with the other half serving as the control group.

To no one's surprise, the screened group had a lot more lung cancer. Because the malignancies were discovered in their very early stages, the patients were immediately put into treatment and showed an excellent survival rate. But, when the data provided by the control group was programmed into the study, it was found that the number of men who died of lung cancer in both the control group and the group diagnosed and treated resulted in virtually identical survival rates.

On the other hand, the early diagnosis and treatment of breast cancer *does* improve the odds for women over the age of fifty, but not for younger women. Under the auspices of the Health Insurance Plan of Greater New York, a 20-year study of 62,000 women (aged 40 to 64) involved offering half the women free annual mammograms and physical examinations, with the other half of the group serving as the control. Far fewer deaths as a result of breast cancer were tabulated in women over age 50 (but not in the younger women) in the group offered free exams than in the control group.

Note: Although no clinical trials have been mounted to determine the usefulness of the vaginal PAP smear, most authorities agree that this test, leading to early diagnosis and treatment, would prove to be of vital importance in increasing survival rates for women.

THE MORTALITY RATE — In 1962, the total cancer mortality rate in the U.S. was 170 persons in every 100,000. In 1982, twenty years later and the latest year for which overall cancer mortality statistics are currently available, the total figure was 185 victims in every 100,000 persons. John Bailar of the Harvard School of Public Health says, "The fundamental problem is not that cancer treatment is ineffective, but that it is not getting better. The figures cited above show why we're worried. Overall cancer mortality is going up."

ANNUAL DEATHS FROM CANCER PER 100 MILLION AMERICANS UNDER AGE 65

Number of Deaths (Male)	Site of Cancer	Number of Deaths (Female)
30,000 25,000 20,000 15,000 10,000 6,000 2,000 0		0 2,000 6,000 10,000 15,000 20,000 25,000 30,000

Legend:
*Nonsmokers
1950s
1960s
1970s

Site of Cancer
Oral Cancer (mouth, esophagus, larynx)
Lung Cancer
Stomach Cancer
Intestines (including rectum)
Liver, Gallbladder & Bile Ducts
Pancreas
Bone
Skin Cancer
Breast Cancer
Bladder
Kidneys
Prostate
Uterine Cancer (cervix)
Uterine Cancer (endometrium)
Uterine Cancer (ovaries)
Brain & Nervous System
Leukemia
Hodgkin's Disease
Other

325

PREVENTION *IS* VITAL — With discouraging statistics like these and the mortality rate from cancer continually creeping upward, there's no question whatsoever but that we must protect ourselves and our loved ones from this killer with every means at our disposal.

FOREWARNED IS FOREARMED

NO ONE CAN DO IT FOR YOU — It has become increasingly obvious that we all have some hard choices to make, but *the guideposts are clearly marked.* You can opt to follow a crooked path with many indulgences and heedless diversions along the way. Or you can examine your lifestyle and decide instead to make whatever changes are necessary to put some of the documented preventives to work for you. It's up to you to choose the road you wish to travel.

Health is the natural state of the body. If you make the right choices *now,* all the evidence promises that the quality of life you can enjoy into your sunset years will be rich with both mental and physical pleasures long past three score years and ten.

Here's to your very good health.

William L. Fischer

For Your Convenience

Most of the consumer products discussed in *How To Fight Cancer And Win* are available in major health food stores nationwide. Always insist on quality products. When purchasing flaxseed (linseed) oil, insist on getting only the **unrefined**, cold-pressed product.

SUGGESTED READING

DIET, NUTRITION, AND CANCER
Committee on Diet, Nutrition, and Cancer
Assembly of Life Sciences, National Research Council
Published By:
National Academy Press
2101 Constitution Avenue NW
Washington, DC 20418

WHAT YOU CAN DO TO PREVENT CANCER
Oliver Alabaster, M.D.
Published By:
Simon & Schuster
1230 Avenue of the Americas
New York, NY 10020

CANCER, RISKS AND PREVENTION
Edited By:
M.P. Vessey, Peofessor of Social & Community Medicine
University of Oxford, and
Muir Gray, Community Physician
Fellow of Green College, University of Oxford
Published By:
Oxford University Press
Walton Street
Oxford, OX2 6DP
Great Britain

**FATS AND OILS - THE COMPLETE GUIDE TO FATS
AND OILS IN HEALTH AND NUTRITION**
Udo Erasmus
Published By:
Alive Books
Vancouver, B.C. V5W 3T1
Canada

THE MACROBIOTIC APPROACH TO CANCER
Garden City Park
Published By:
Avery, 1991

RESOURCE REFERENCES

LIVINGSTON THERAPY
Livingston Foundation Medical Center
3232 Duke Street
San Diego, CA 92110
Phone: 619-224-3515

GERSON METHOD
The Gerson Institute
P.O. Box 430
Bonita, CA 92002
Phone: 619-267-1150

MACROBIOTIC INSTITUTE
Kushi Institute
P.O. Box 7
Becket, MA 01233
Phone: 413-623-5742

HYDRAZINE SULFATE INFORMATION:
Dr. Joseph Gold
Syracuse Research Institute
600 East Genesee Street
Syracuse, NY 13202
Phone 315-472-6616

GREEN TEA
Wah Ying Hong Enterprises
232 Canal Street
New York, NY 10013
Phone 212-941-8954
(Available at most Health Food stores)

GLOSSARY

Abscisic acid: a kind of plant hormone which inhibits the growth of plants. Counteracts growth-promoting substances.

Cancer cell: a cell which has somehow escaped normal controls over growth and division. Cancer begins with a single cell which produces clones of itself (called daughter cells) which invade adjacent tissues and ofter interferes with their normal activity. Cancer cells have abnormal glucose requirements and produce lactic acid, which puts an extra burden on the liver. Cells which proliferate but stay together form benign tumors, not cancers. Those cells which disperse through the blood or lymph are called malignant, or cancerous cells.

Cancer: a disease, or group of diseases, characterized by a loss of cellular control mechanisms, the invasion of surrounding tissues and a strong tendency to metastasize (migrate) to distant sites. Cancer may recur even after attempted removal and cause the death of the patient, unless adequately treated.

Carcinogen: any factor, but mainly synthetic chemicals, that is capable of transforming a normal cell into a cancerous one.

Carcinomas: malignant tumors arising in cells of epithelial origin. Encompassing most breast, lung, liver, etc. tumors, they are the most common type of cancer.

Carotene: yellow or orange pigments commonly found in plants, which can be converted into Vitamin A in the liver.

Cartilage: the most important connective tissue of the human skeleton after bone. Contains glycoproteins but lacks blood vessels and nerves.

Chemotherapy: the use of drugs, and especially of cytotoxic agents, in the treatment of cancer and other diseases.

Chlorophyll: a green pigment found in algae and most higher plants, which is responsible for capturing light in the process of photosynthesis.

DNA: deoxyribonucleic acid. Double-stranded molecule that forms the genetic material of all cells and many viruses.

Enzymes: protein catalysts which are responsible for the high rate and the specificity of most biochemical reactions. Higher forms of life are inconceivable without enzymes.

Essential fatty acids: substances required in the diet for normal growth. These include linoleic and linolenic acids.

Folic acid: a water-soluable vitamin of the B-complex involved in many enzymatic reactions.

Free radicals: an atom or atom group which carries an unpaired electron but no charge. Free radicals are very short-lived but can cause serious damage to living tissues. They are counteracted by reff radical scavengers, such as Vitamin C.

Gene: the smallest physical unit of heredity normally found in a cell.

Interferons: proteins produced by virally-infected cells, as well as by non-infected white blood cells, which are able to prevent the further replication of viruses.

Interleukins: factors involved in communication among white blood cells. May also be produced by some non-white blood cells. Involved in activating t-cells and in making macrophages (scavenger cells) more effective. Interleukin-2 (IL-2) is used in the treatment of kidney cancer, melanoma and other tumors, but is highly toxic and rarely curative.

Leukemia: a malignant overproduction of white blood cells, which crowds out normal red blood cells and destroys platelet production. Death results mainly from indirect effects of this process.

Leukocytes: blood cells which have a nucleus, but lack hemoglobin. Includes several categories: granulocytes whose granules are visible under the microscope and a granulocytes (including both lymphocytes and monocytes).

Lipids: a broad category of organic compounds including fats, waxes, steroids, the fat-soluable vitamins (A, D, E, K), prostaglandins, carotenes and chlorophylls.

Lipoprotein: a mixture of protein and lipids important in may biological reactions.

Lymph: clear fluid found in the vessels of the lymphatic system. Responsible for returning proteins from the tissue fluid to the blood.

Macrophage: scavenger (phagocytic) cell of connective tissue not usuallyfound in the blood. The two main types are (1) the wandering macrophages and (2) the static macrophages, which migrate to the site of an infection and engulf foreign particles.

Metabolism: the sum of all chemical and physical processes in a living body. More specifically, the term can refer to the combined action of a body's enzymes.

Metastasis: movement of cancer cells from a primary growth to a distant site, usually via the blood or lymph. Secondary growths in vital organs can be more dangerous than the primary tumor.

Myeloma: a malignant cancer of the bone marrow (myeloid) tissue. Causes anemia as its major symptom and mainly affects middle-aged and elderly persons.

Oncologist: a medical doctor who specializes in the treatment of cancer, especially through the use of chemotherapy.

Oncology: the science which studies the disease process of cancer.

Peptide: two or more amino acids linked together by a peptide bond. Long chains of peptides are usually called polypeptides.

Polysaccharide: a carbohydrate which, although somewhat like a sugar, lacks a sweet taste. Some examples are cellulose, starch and glycogen.

Prostaglandins: fatty acid derivatives which are continuously produced by many cells. Released into the blood stream like hormones, but unlike hormones only effective over short distances.

Pulmonary: relating to the lung.

Sarcoma: a malignant tumor arising in tissues of mesenchymal origin, such as connective tissue, bone, cartilage or striated muscle.

Syndrome: the signs and symptoms associated with a disease, which taken together constitute a picture of that disease.

T-cell: a lymphocyte formed in the bone marrow which then travels to the thymus for 'processing,' where it learns to recognize 'self' from 'non-self.' The t-cell then travels on to the spleen and lymph nodes. Some t-cells assist B- cells, others stimulate macrophages, while yet others suppress immune responses.

Toxicity: the state of being poisonous.

Virus: a minute infectious agent which is unable to multiply by itself, but can do so by using a living cell as its host. A virus can pass through the smallest bacterial filter and can only be seen with an elecron microscope.

Vitamin A: A fat-soluble vitamin, the lack of which affects all tissues, but mostly the eyes. Infants and children are especially susceptible to vitamin A deficiencies.

Vitamin B complex: a group of 12 water-soluble vitamins, including biotin, cyanocobalamin, folic acid, nicotinic acid, pantothenic acid, pyridoxine and riboflavin.

Vitamin C: ascorbic acid. A water soluble sugar acid, which is especially abundant in fruit and tomatoes. Can be destroyed by cooking. Complete absence results in scurvy. Appears to have an important role in cancer prevention and possibly treatment.

Vitamin D: a small group of fat-soluble vitamins, deficiency of which causes the disease rickets. Can be synthesized in the skin by exposure to ultraviolet light or if necessary supplemented in the diet with fish liver oil. Required for healthy bone and teeth.

Vitamin E: A group of fat-soluble vitamins obtained from seed oils, wheat germ, etc. Deficiency causes infertility and kidney degeneration.

Vitamin K: fat-soluble vitamins required for syntheses in the liver of a substance required for blood clotting. Produced by many plants and microorganisms, including some normally found in the gut.

Vitamin: an organic substance that is not normally made by an animal but has to be obtained from the environment in tiny amounts. Lack of a vitamin generally results in a specific deficiency disease.

INDEX

INDEX

INDEX

Great Pharmacopoeia - 187
Green Tea - 55, 56

H

Hagiwara, Dr. Yoshihide - 68
Hanna, Michael G. - 33
Ha-ras gene - 224
Harris, Dr. Curtis - 5
Hartman, Dr. Ernst - 225
Health Maintenance Organizations (HMOs) - 36
heredity and cancer - 224
Hernuss, Dr. Peter - 180
Hirsch, Dr. J. - 115
Hodgkin's Disease - 23, 47, 146
Hoover, H.C. - 33
Hoppe-Seyler, Ernst F. - 119
hydrazine sulfate - 29, 319
hydrogenation - 96
hypertension- 149
hyperthermia - 31, 301

I

immune system - 26, 222, 227
immunotherapy - 27, 30, 72, 290
immunotoxins - 32, 33
India (fat studies) - 141
interferon - 27
interleukin - 2, 26
irradiated foods - 247
iron - 267
Issels, Dr. Josef - 299-303

J

Johnson, Noel - 178, 181

K

Karmali, Dr. Rashida, A. - 106
Kelly, Dr. William - 303-306
kidney cancer - 10, 11, 48, 205
Knudson, Dr. A.G. - 223
Kohler, Heinz - 33

Koprowski, Dr. Hilary - 32
Korchemny, Remi - 181
Kremer, Dr. Joel M. - 106
Kromhout, D. - 104
Kushi, Michic - 188

L

laetrile - 210-212, 277
Lands, Dr. William - 107
laryngeal cancer - 8, 10
laser surgery - 30
lead - 242
Lebedow - 119
lecithin - 94, 101, 118, 272-274
Lenormand, Dr. E. - 180
leukemia - 28, 31, 32, 47
Liebig, Baron Justus von - 119
linoleic acid - 59, 72, 101, 105, 109, 112, 117, 120, 126, 137, 139, 140, 157, 254, 274
linolenic acid - 60, 72, 101, 105, 108, 110, 112, 117, 137, 139, 140, 157, 234, 254, 274
linseed oil - 109, 117-163, 215, 234
linseed oil diet - 152-157
Liotta, Dr. Lance - 2
lipophilic molecules - 29
liver cancer - 10, 11, 33, 83, 216
Livingston, Dr. Virginia - 74-77
Los Alamos National Laboratory - 44
lumpectomy - 42
lung cancer - 8, 10, 15, 23, 30, 57, 209, 224, 255, 324
lymphatic system - 6, 12, 16, 133, 146
lymphoma - 30, 31

M

macrobiotic diet - 18, 186-198
macrophages - 26, 28, 206
maitake mushroom - 55

338

INDEX

INDEX

INDEX OF CHARTS AND ILLUSTRATIONS

OTHER OUTSTANDING BOOKS
ON HEALTH AND NATURAL HEALING
FROM FISCHER PUBLISHING

**Secrets To A Healthy Heart And Low Cholesterol
by William L. Fischer**

This book can be your valued partner in lowering or maintaining your cholesterol level. Learn about cholesterol, what it does, how it works and why too much is dangerous. It shows you how to take positive steps in improving your current situation and maintaining it for life long health. Hardening of the arteries, or atherosclerosis, is also discussed in detail. It gives no warning signals until it is almost too late. There are effective measures you can take to help delay, prevent and reverse this very serious health problem. Included is also the world famous scientific breakthrough formula by Prof. Norgaard, M.D., D.D.S. from Denmark that has helped thousands of people overcome their illnesses.

ISBN 0-915421-13-5 ....$14.95

**Mysterious Cause Of Illness and How To Overcome Every Disease From Constipation to Cancer
by Jonn Matsen, N.D.**

Famed Canadian doctor uncovers the mysterious *REAL* cause of illness—and shows you how to overcome every disease from constipation to cancer. Dr. Matsen's acclaimed food-based "miracle cures" use *no* drugs, *no* surgery. They simply turn on the natural "internal healing power" built into every human body. Here is a safe, easy approach to health and longevity that has cured many "hopeless" cases after conventional medicine has failed! If you read nothing else, read Dr. Matsen's new revelations of secret remedies.

ISBN 0-915421-09-7 .... $18.95

343

Eye Secrets To Better Sight
by William L. Fischer

This important new book discusses the latest natural treatments for most common eye diseases. The author presents symptoms of various eye conditions from cataracts and glaucoma to macular degeneration, from the rare to the common place. He describes the warning signs of numerous eye problems and how to cope with them successfully. Also covered is the very latest in medical technology and explains how new procedures can cure most common sight defects forever. A must to read for everyone who cares about their eyesight—your window to the world—and that of your loved ones.

ISBN 0-915421-14-3 ....$18.95

The Romance Of Creative Healthy Cookery
by William and Trudy Fischer

We know you'll fall in love with this book because over 800,000 European women with osteoporosis-type conditions have already greatly benefited. All of the recipes are time-tested and medically endorsed. These new inventive dishes were created by health minded experts and nutritionally oriented chefs and have been adapted for ingredients that can be easily purchased at your local grocery store. The book includes calcium-rich recipes to fight or prevent osteoporosis, nutritious meals for the whole family, budget dishes fit for royalty and think light...cook light...eat light recipes everybody will enjoy.

ISBN 0-915421-11-9 ....$18.95

How To Fight Cancer And Win by William L. Fischer

It clearly spells out real cancer preventives and cures, many never before published, with strong scientific documentation and stories of miraculous cures. They are all presented in a concise, easy-to-understand style. You can put this vast knowledge into practice to ensure that this deadly disease never strikes home.

ISBN 0-915421-18-6 . . . . $29.97
Hardcover. Newly revised, updated edition.

Breakthrough In Arthritis
by William Fischer

If you thought there was nothing you could do for your painful condition, you need to read this book and discover freedom from arthritic pain. Learn more about the complex of nearly one hundred often crippling diseases called arthritis, such as rheumatism, bursitis, gout, carpel tunnel syndrome and more. Sound, natural, safe remedies are offered in detail. Also described in this book is the newest breakthrough formula of a leading world authority on arthritic pain.

ISBN 0-915421-15-1 . . . .$18.95

Miraculous Breakthroughs for Prostate and Impotency Problems
by William L. Fischer

Good news for every man who has prostate or occasional impotency problems. This new book describes in detail many of the latest therapeutic discoveries from Europe and America that can prevent, relieve or cure prostate disease, without the agony of prostate surgery. The book also discusses other male problems like testicle diseases, cancer, and the subject of impotency with honesty and sensitivity.

ISBN 0-915421-12-7 . . . .$18.95

The Miracle Healing Power Through Nature's Pharmacy by William L. Fischer

In *Miracle Healing Power Through Nature's Pharmacy*, you'll learn how to use nature's herb medicines to treat: *arthritis, rheumatism, sprains, strains, gout, colds and influenza, coughs, sinusitis, bronchitis, asthma, high blood pressure, poor circulation, hardening of the arteries, high cholesterol, headaches, ulcers, prostate problems, varicose veins, diabetes, stress, depression, insomnia, menopausal syndrome* and much, much more.

This complete and most natural healing system is now available to you. You will learn how easy it is to make herbal hot and cold infusions and decoctions (teas), ointments, compresses, poultices, and tinctures. Read this extraordinary book and prove it to yourself. You will be surprisingly amazed at the unexpected wonderful results!

ISBN 0-915421-04-6 . . . . $19.95

The Youth Renewal Revolution by Alexander Woodward

Renewed youth... a longer life... a surge of healthy vitality... the discoveries and breakthroughs that make it all possible... all organized into one of the most brilliant plans ever created for people who are ready for rejuvenation *right now!* Just look at the benefits that this breakthrough book holds for you: Eliminate wrinkles, renew sexual energy, lose weight, rejuvenate, renew youth. Don't let another day go by, robbing you of your youth and vitality... Join the youth renewal revolution!

ISBN 0-915421-17-8 . . . . $12.95

Shipping/Handling $4.00 for one book.
Additional books $1.00 each

Fischer Publishing
P.O. Box 368
Canfield, Ohio 44406
(216) 533-1232